DRAMA SCRIPTS
FOR PEOPLE WITH
SPECIAL NEEDS

T0329510

DRAMA SCRIPTS
FOR PEOPLE WITH
SPECIAL NEEDS

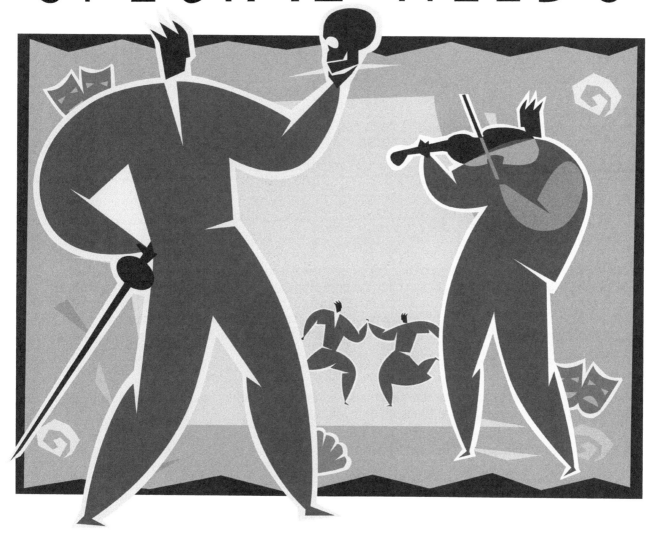

SHEREE VICKERS

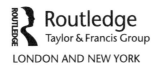

Routledge
Taylor & Francis Group

LONDON AND NEW YORK

For Tybalt

Group members are referred to as 'he' and the group
facilitator as 'she' in the text, for purposes of clarity alone

First published 2005 by Speechmark Publishing Ltd.

Published 2017 by Routledge
2 Park Square, Milton Park, Abingdon, Oxon OX14 4RN
711 Third Avenue, New York, NY 10017, USA

Routledge is an imprint of the Taylor & Francis Group, an informa business

Copyright © Sheree Vickers, 2005
Illustrations by Joanne Miles

British Library Cataloguing in Publication Data

Vickers, Sheree
    Drama scripts for people with special needs : inclusive drama
    for PMLD, autistic spectrum and special neess groups.
    – (A Speechmark creative groupwork resource)
    1. Drama in education 2. People with disabilities – Education
    3. Drama – Therapeutic use
    I. Title
    371.9'04466

ISBN 9780863885297 (pbk)

CONTENTS

ACKNOWLEDGEMENTS

Sarah Watney for reteaching me the value of song, and for all her help in planning the early special needs workshops.

The pupils and teachers at Manor Green School (formerly Catherington) for providing such a rich, exciting and friendly environment.

POLKA Theatre for Children, for introducing me to special needs drama work and allowing me to include workshops developed for their Arts Access programme.

Flo Longhorn for her unique publications and continued support in this sensory quest.

Richard Burbage at Paddock School for his honesty, dedication and enthusiasm.

The helpers, carers and participants at Merton Crossroads for their humour during our 'Jack and the Beanstalk' rehearsals.

Zoe Maxine for setting the standard in drama assistance, and, last but not least, my husband, for his acceptance of the bizarre props and unusual costumes that continue to clutter up our house!

INTRODUCTION

This book contains a drama toolkit of adaptable scripts, workshop breakdowns and activities. Its aim is to build confidence in those wanting to use drama with their particular group of people with special needs, or, for those already experienced, to inspire them with a library of ideas designed to assist their creative lessons.

Each script has been fully worked with groups of varying ages and abilities, and often includes notes of experience – documenting sessions where the unexpected happened and how it was handled. As with any group of people with special needs, getting to know their needs is paramount in order to plan the drama for their specific requirements. However, the scripts and workshop breakdowns included in this book are guaranteed to work even at a first meeting.

A few notes before starting the drama

Begin and end each drama session with a related song, poem or activity. This 'bookends' the drama nicely and is important as it helps to establish what is 'playtime' and what is real. Any song or poem will do, but the Explanation of Activities chapter contains various suggestions, including Copy Mime Circle, Freeze As and a suggested Opening Meet and Greet Song or Goodbye Song. A short discussion just prior to the final song, poem or activity is also beneficial as it gives the group members a chance to discuss what they enjoyed (or didn't) about the drama, which is useful feedback for you in planning future sessions. Preparation is vital for a successful workshop.

If visiting a group for the first time, try and arrange a preliminary meeting to discuss individual needs; look at the space to be used and talk about expectations. Limit the number of group members to between 6 and 12. Although this is not always possible, I find this bracket an ideal number as it provides both a personal and collective drama experience. The drama sessions themselves should be no longer than one hour. Any more than this without a break and the group (not to mention the leader) can get very tired.

To start planning any drama workshop, brainstorm and write down any ideas that come to mind. These notes are a good reference point should the workshop turn out to be inappropriate, or in need of modification for another group with different needs.

When working with a group over multiple sessions, one approach is to spend the first lesson leading the group through the entire drama (although this is not always possible with longer dramas such as the 'Macbeth' workshop breakdown). This may feel like a whirlwind trip, but can give the group an idea of what to expect. Each future session is then spent recapping and breaking the drama down, exploring and developing each stage of the journey more deeply. Another approach is to discover the drama slowly, keeping the group in suspense as the story gains momentum.

If the group is particularly nervous or needs additional sensory guidance, introduce the props and costumes for the drama beforehand, passing them around for the participants to touch and explore while discussing what characters might use them. Spend a preliminary session dressing up as these characters and practising key phrases of dialogue, incorporating (if available) electronic communication devices or vocal aids. Aside from building confidence, this process also helps to gain group members' permission to participate in the drama. This is important: asking a simple question, such as 'Would you like to meet them?' or 'Should we go and see what they're up to?', and accepting the answer (see the 'Professor Wafflepuff' script for further advice on what to do when the answer is 'No') helps to empower the participants' decision-making and places value on their choices.

Avoid wearing busy or bright clothing as it can distract the participants. Tie long hair away, wear minimal jewellery and no perfume as it can interfere with the senses you are trying to stimulate.

Start building a 'drama box' full of useful props and costumes. Some handy props include a mirror, feathers, confetti, a water spray bottle, soft balls, balloons, animal snap cards (see the Explanation of Activities chapter for ways to use these), different coloured scarves and music to dance to. Start to explore textures by rubbing different materials against your cheeks and the back of your hand. This helps you to discover their sensation and was how I discovered that bubble-wrap makes an ideal whale!

Setting up the space

A circle is the traditional formation for a drama session, using either mats or chairs to define the space. This initial circle is also a safety mechanism, giving the group a visual grounding to come back to should the drama take an unexpected turn. It also provides a space for some to watch the drama, if the idea of joining in is too overwhelming.

> **NOTE:** Don't be afraid to stop the drama at any time and come back to this formation. It often helps to review the drama and reiterate that it is pretend. This can be important if the group is scared or confused by changing roles or if you feel the drama is getting too off track.

For a group with limited mobility, or in a limited space, keep the participants in a circle and bring the drama to them. If the group is used to working in a particular arrangement, for example a traditional classroom setting, there is nothing to stop you from continuing to use this formation, adapting the drama to the space available.

A large hall is wonderful to play in. It can provide space to explore the marketplace in 'Jack and the Beanstalk' (with different stands in different corners) or to create an ice-skating rink on a beautiful frozen lake. However, as a new or large space may upset some participants, still define the circle/safe area as mentioned above, possibly having it in one corner of the hall.

If you are preparing a workshop for presentation, practise in the presentation space as much as possible. Define a backstage area with chairs for participants to return to, show them the area where you can be found during the performance and mark points on the stage with tape as 'visual cues' for the cast to stand on to say their lines.

Presentation rather than performance

In traditional theatre, the job of the actor is to create a memorable experience for the audience. When using drama as a learning tool, the emphasis should be on creating a memorable experience for the participants. I don't discourage the showing of work, as it is an extremely valuable way of giving a group a sense of purpose and challenge. The rewards are tremendous for those that perform; however, the sense of failure for those that can't, can be equally immense. This is why I deliberately don't use the words performance or actor. There should be no sense of guilt attached to those who do not wish to stand up in front of an audience.

I have substituted the word performance with presentation, and actor with participant. Group members can participate in the drama even if it is only during the rehearsal stage. Alternatively, they might feel empowered to take on the role of playing the background music or opening the curtains. All of these roles within the drama are invaluable and should be treated as such; hence, if a curtain call is required (and it invariably is), give these background participants their own acknowledgement. In presentations involving those with profound and multiple learning difficulties (PMLD), the emphasis should still be on giving participants a worthwhile experience, and there is nothing more fascinating to watch than a staged drama workshop.

Please don't act

As mentioned, the role of the teacher or leader within the workshops is not to direct or act, but to facilitate a dramatic experience for the group. The aim is to demonstrate roles within the script, not to show off acting skills. Actually, full-blown performing is to be discouraged as it can overwhelm the group and remember, you are there for their experience, not your own!

The best way to describe this facilitating is to think of a ringleader in the circus. A ringleader has the freedom to observe the action or interact within the drama, taking on various responsibilities as necessary. Even in a presentation situation with an audience watching, there's nothing to stop you from leading the drama in this way. During one memorable presentation we even had the audience sing the Opening Meet and Greet Song with us!

> **NOTE:** Personally I love including the audience in drama presentations, for example, if using 'The Operation' script for a presentation, have the doctor ask the audience the question 'Do we need this?'

Taking on a role

Roleplay is an extremely powerful tool. It allows participants to make choices, exploring situations and relationships with an emotional safety net. It is not them making mistakes, but their character within the drama.

The objective of taking on a role is either to move the drama forward or to demonstrate that particular role before the participants present it themselves. Demonstrating can be as simple as saying 'I'm going to put this coat on and say "Dear me!" Would you like to have a go?' This process of demonstration can be repeated as often as necessary.

If casting for a presentation, add an extra role for yourself. For example, in the 'Training Day' script, cast the Postman from the group and have yourself as an assistant to help guide, with questions such as 'Shall we train them up now? Shall I go and see if McHungry is ready for his/her letter now?', etc.

Dropping role is just as simple. By removing the visual cue of the hat or coat, you can resume any needed teacher or leader duties before returning to the drama. The participants never perceive this 'stepping outside of' or 'dropping role' as wrong or inappropriate, and it is a good way to observe the group's responses, to guide them further, or to deal with any problems as they may occur.

Occasionally members of the group can get very nervous at the thought of meeting a new character. Before introducing the role, return to the circle and ask them to choose the character's costume. Add a bit of humour by getting confused about how the costume should be worn, for example, if they suggest wearing a cape around your neck, put it around your waist asking 'Is this my neck? No? So where is my neck then?' Repeat this process with other parts of the body. Get them to continue building the character by deciding if the voice should be loud or quiet. Ask them what sort of things your character might say before telling them you are going to practise. Having the group make each character decision will usually stop any apprehension. Return to the drama by reiterating that it is pretend and asking them if they'd like to pretend with you.

NOTE: For a full breakdown on introducing a scary character, see the 'Dragon Sleep' script.

A note on using puppets

Groups respond very well to puppets. Participants who have difficulty in making eye contact will often engage fully with a puppet. They are also a good way to explore cause and effect. For example, putting a finger in the puppet's eye will hurt the puppet and therefore demonstrate safely that it's not a good thing to do. Even the sound of a puppet's speech gagging when fingers are shoved into its mouth helps to illustrate this. Another benefit is that it allows you to continue the drama while keeping one eye focused on the group.

Time often needs to be spent introducing the concept of a puppet. Don't worry if the drama stops while the group members explore where the hand goes, how the mouth moves, even passing the puppet around for them all to explore. If the puppet is too much of a distraction first time around, put it away and carry on with the drama as another character. When I first introduced the Goosey puppet in 'Jack and the Beanstalk', there was a lot of excitement and some participants were even scared of him. However, over the four weeks of workshops, I gradually reintroduced him and the group became very protective of both the character and the actual puppet.

Puppets don't have to be elaborate. Finger puppets, a simple sock with stuck-on eyes, or even a picture on a stick can be used. In fact, picture sticks are great to give to each participant playing a particular character. Best of all, you don't need to be a master puppeteer to use them.

And finally

None of these scripts or workshop breakdowns need to be learnt word-perfect, and they can be worked through with the pages in front of you. However, any text or story presented in a bland way will be uninspiring for the pupils, not to mention yourself. Energy and fun are the key to any drama session.

Continually repeat dialogue and use the participants' names as often as possible to help personalise the drama. Don't rush, as individuals with special needs often have slower reaction times. Repeat key phrases, their names, any sensory stimulus and allow time for participants to respond.

Learn to adapt your vocabulary. Replacing phrases such as 'No, that's wrong' with 'That's an interesting choice' or 'I've never seen it done like that before' will help to value their decisions and may even develop drama possibilities not even considered!

Sometimes the group will want to discuss things that are not related to the workshop. Stopping them from doing so could make them feel as if their ideas in general are not valued, but at the same time, they shouldn't get too distracted from the drama. Therefore, other stock phrases can include 'Thanks for telling me' or 'Can you remember that and tell me later?' Alternatively, if the distraction is too major for them to be able to participate fully, give the problem over to a helper. (This also applies for any traumas related to taking on a role, as mentioned earlier.)

Over the years, when leading drama workshops, having helpers to keep an eye on the participants for any problems or to join in and encourage individuals has been my most valuable resource. Discuss with regular carers or helpers what they would like their role within the drama to be (passive observer or fully interactive participant) and ask their advice on the best way of informing you of potential problems during the workshop. (I have often been unaware of a participant needing changing or having a seizure because the carer has handled it perfectly.) When visiting a group, conflicts do sometimes arise.

Occasionally I have had altercations with people who have had very specific ideas about what drama should be and how a group should be managed. Try and commit them to your way of leading the workshop and allow for a feedback or follow-up time, as no contradictions should occur during the drama session.

Lastly, don't panic if all goes disastrously wrong. One very memorable catastrophe of my own involved a group of autistic boys: I was assured they were very capable and I discovered the opposite to be true. They were unprepared for a new environment and I was just unprepared. All I remember is coming away from that session with future knowledge of what not to do!

It is all a learning curve, and remember, there are no absolutes in drama. No right or wrong. Just endless choices. So have fun!

SCRIPTS

Most drama scripts are rehearsed and performed as written. These scripts however, have been especially designed to provide a structure to play around in. They (and the Explanation of Activities chapter) are the basis of your drama toolkit.

Combine the two to create different adventures, for example befriending the dragon in 'Dragon Sleep' can be adapted and used in a workshop on 'Hamlet' and meeting his father's ghost. For more sensory dramas, strip the language away completely to use only key phrases, sounds or textures.

Although they can be rehearsed and performed as written, these scripts are adaptable for infinite dramas with whatever you or your group's imagination offer, and they can be combined with the additional activities suggested to provide enough scope to develop ideas for a lifetime.

Despite the small character lists, the material is for whole-group participation, and it allows for spontaneous interactions. Don't be afraid to improvise. The script is your safety net to fall back on should improvisations become too distracting or uncontrolled.

Drama allows us to practise, teaching us how to handle situations in life. Although the lessons may be the same, they never feel repetitive when taught within a different context or story.

TRAINING DAY

This basic format trains the group in a chosen profession, even allowing participants to go out on assignment before gaining their qualifications.

It was first worked with a group of 7–10-year-olds with severe speech language difficulties as part of POLKA Theatre's Curtain-Up Scheme for their 2003 production of 'Martha's Wild Goose Chase'.

Props List

- Post bag
- Whistle
- 'Heavy' box
- 'Fragile' box
- 'Urgent' box
- 'Certificate of Achievement' documents for each participant (see template included)
- Four letters (marked with 'Must Be Delivered By Hand') for the various 'Mc' characters listed above
- Activities for each letter
- Costume box (if a box containing different hats, wigs and materials is not available, explore each character's facial expressions and sounds, for example, 'I wonder what this character would say or look like?')

Character List

- Postman
- McSnooty
- McSmelly
- McHungry
- McMeany

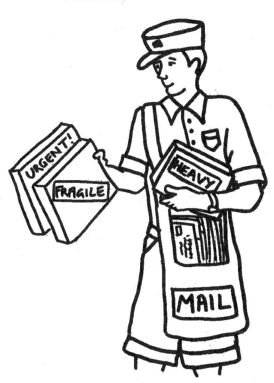

THE SCRIPT

POSTMAN: Hello everyone. Do you know what I do? Can you guess?

Spend some time looking at the postbag, costume box and other props and take suggestions on your profession from the group.

> **NOTE:** Suggested characters may include Father Christmas or even a burglar. Accept all of these before steering the group back to who you actually are, acknowledging those who may have guessed correctly.

POSTMAN: Well, I could be all of those things, but in fact, I'm a postman. I deliver letters and parcels to people, and I'm here today to train you all to be postmen or postwomen. Would you all like to help me to deliver the mail?

> **NOTE:** Some participants may suddenly decide that they want to be something completely different, for example, an elephant! If this happens, let them be an elephant who just happens to deliver the mail! Alternatively, if they can't be persuaded otherwise, allow them to indulge in their elephant fantasy, and watch while you continue to train the others.

POSTMAN: Now this training is very important. We have to learn how to:
  - carry a very heavy package

Demonstrate either with mime and/or a very large box with 'Heavy' written across it.

  - carry a very delicate package

A box with 'Fragile' written across it and possibly something inside it that makes a rattling sound.

  - deliver an urgent package

A box with 'Urgent' written across it that has to be carried quickly across the space.

- and also how to run away from a dog.

Looking scared, run and hide while you or a helper make barking noises – this particular training exercise can be followed with the whistle and tea break call to bring back some order to the group – see below.

> **NOTE:** Running away from the dog developed as a bit of fun one day and turned into a mini-drama itself. Some group members wanted to try and befriend the dog, whereas others wanted to scare it away. I ended up casting myself as the dog and had a wonderful helper guide the group into interaction with the dog. It turned out that the dog 'just wanted to be fed' because it was hungry and after that it was a very friendly dog indeed! See the 'Dragon Sleep' script for a sample breakdown of this interaction.

POSTMAN: ... and if I blow the whistle it is time for a tea break and we have to run back to our places as quickly as possible and sit down. Shall we practise doing that?

Ask the group members to stand up and, on the count of three, blow the whistle and shout 'Tea Break' so that they can practise running back to their places.

POSTMAN: Excellent! Now let's get on with the training ...

Randomly call out the training exercises listed above and have the group members (either as individuals or all together) demonstrate them. Call for a tea break at any time. When you feel that sufficient training has been completed, ask the group members to sit down, ready for their first assignment.

> **NOTE:** Some members of the group might take the training literally and ask for either stamps or a real postbox. Remind them that they are training and that they are only 'pretending'.

POSTMAN: Now the next part of the training involves actually delivering a letter.

Take a letter out of the postbag.

POSTMAN: The first letter is for McSnooty. Uh, oh! Have you heard about McSnooty?

Get the costume box out and explore the clothes.

POSTMAN: What do you think McSnooty looks like? Would he wear a hat/shirt/coat like this?

Start to build up the costume and personality.

Routledge
Taylor & Francis Group

POSTMAN: What sort of things do you think McSnooty might say? Who would like to be McSnooty?

Cast and dress McSnooty and place him on a chair in front of the group.

POSTMAN: Now who thinks they're brave enough to deliver the letter?

Choose someone.

POSTMAN: Remember, this letter has to be delivered by hand.

Refer to the 'Must Be Delivered By Hand' message on the envelope.

POSTMAN: You can't just throw the letter at McSnooty or put it in the letterbox. You must actually give it to him. OK, good luck!

> **NOTE:** If no one would like to be the character, then take the role on yourself. 'Shall I be McSnooty? Who's going to deliver the letter to me?' (See 'Please Don't Act' in the Introduction for more on adopting roles.)

Get the group to wish the Postman good luck and guide them into delivering the letter by hand. You may even want to remind them to knock on the door or ring the bell.

> **NOTE:** Often a spontaneous interaction between the Postman and the 'Mc' character can take place. It's usually a lovely bit of improvised dialogue, but on the odd occasion where it becomes unnecessarily negative or nasty, stop the drama, reassess and possibly replay the scene. For example, 'As postal workers we have to be polite. We're not allowed to be nasty to people. So how could we redeliver the letter, but this time being nice?'

POSTMAN: Wonderful! I wonder what's inside the letter. Shall we open it and have a look?

Open the envelope and discover instructions for a game or activity inside. It could be as simple as 'Sing a song' or 'Play musical statues' or (in the case of McSmelly), 'Name three things that smell really bad'. Each of these activities can be repeated by different individuals or the whole group for as long as seems appropriate, before moving on to the next letter. (See Explanation of Activities chapter for a description of various games.)

POSTMAN: The next letter is for Mc _____ . Uh, oh! Have you heard about

Mc _____ ?

Repeat the process above for as many of the script characters (McSmelly, McHungry, McMeany) as you want.

> **NOTE:** Occasionally a character may not want to open his letter and you will need to reassure him that it is OK and be very persuasive. On one occasion, I wasn't watching closely, and the character actually ate the letter! We just assumed that a lovely cake had been sent and moved on to the next character (making sure the group was clear that this letter was not to be eaten).

Once all the letters have been delivered, blow the whistle for a tea break and finish the training.

POSTMAN: Congratulations. You have all passed the training and are now fully qualified postal workers.

Give each group member a Certificate of Achievement (see p18), shake their hands and congratulate them individually by name.

Further ideas for a sensory workshop

- Pass around objects of different sizes, shapes and weights for the first part of the training.

- Brush some furry material across participants' legs and arms for the dog.

- Actually have some tea at tea break time.

- As well as the activities in each letter, have a smelly letter for McSmelly, a silvery glamorous letter for McSnooty, a cake for McHungry and something that needs to be divided for McMeany (so that the character of McMeany needs to be persuaded to share with the group).

- Add some song and music for travelling to deliver each letter, for example, to the tune of 'The Bear Went Over The Mountain':

    We're off to deliver a letter, a letter, a letter.
    We're off to deliver a letter, I hope that they are home.
    We knock upon the door. We knock upon the door.
    We're here to deliver a letter, a letter, a letter.
    We're here to deliver a letter and then we can go home.

- End by dressing the group up as postal workers and showing them their new look in a mirror.

Additional games and activities

- 'Delivering The Mail' game (see the Explanation of Activities chapter).

- Have a party to celebrate your new qualifications.

- Each delivery could be a journey in itself. For example, to a cold climate, or on a plane, or by boat to where these different people live. (See the 'My Neighbourhood' script for one example of a journey.)

- Discover more about each of the characters who receives a letter. For example, what does McHungry do?

- Create parcels for different countries and spend time discovering what people in these countries might want or need. Take a drama journey to these countries to deliver the parcels. Listen to different world music to accompany each delivery, asking 'Where do you think we're going today?'

- Make a postbox and deliver letters to each other in the group, or arrange an actual trip to the post office or postbox to send a real letter.

Alternative scenarios for future dramas

Super-hero training school

'I'm a Super-Hero. I help to rescue people and keep law and order.'

The training activities could include striking a heroic pose and getting changed quickly. (If stuck for ideas, ask the group for suggestions on what they might need to learn to do.) The assignment could involve helping various characters in trouble. For example, an old lady and a cat: 'My cat is stuck in a tree, can you all meow like a cat to try and get her down?'

Going to sea

'I'm the captain of a sailing ship and I'm here to train you all as sailors.'

The training activities could include scrubbing the decks, hoisting the sails and saying 'Aye aye Captain' while saluting. The assignment could involve going to sea and meeting various characters, for example, a mermaid or a whale. (Extend this drama with the 'Under the Sea' workshop breakdown.)

A lovely way of ending this particular drama could be giving out medals for bravery, hard work, seamanship, etc.

On a building site

'I'm the foreman on a building site and I'm here to train you all up as builders.'

The activities could involve bricklaying, hammering, fixing the electricity, painting, etc, while the characters could be different people needing different houses, for example a dog kennel, a palace for a princess, or a bigger shell for a tortoise.

> **NOTE:** Regardless of the characters or situation used in this script, always keep the tea break whistle-blow as it is an ideal way of restoring focus.

Routledge
Taylor & Francis Group

✻ Certificate of Achievement ✻

This is to certify that

has successfully completed the

Training Day Requirements

and is now a fully qualified

Signed

Dated

THE OPERATION

This basic format is ideal for exploring what is right and wrong, and it can be adapted to teach almost any subject. This particular script teaches the group some of the vital organs in the human body.

Props List

- Nurse's hat or badge

- Medical checklist (see p25) and a pen

- Doctor's coat and toy stethoscope

- Picture props of some of the body's vital organs, for example heart, stomach, lungs, brain and liver

- A wall chart labelled 'Vital Organs of the Body' with matching pictures of the vital organs to be used in the drama

- Pins to stick the corresponding picture props onto the chart

- A collection of silly objects to pull out of the patient's stomach, for example a model car, a banana, a teddy bear, etc

- Table and sheet or a chair

- A box marked 'No'

Character List

Doctor Bumblebee

Nurse Able

Patient(s)

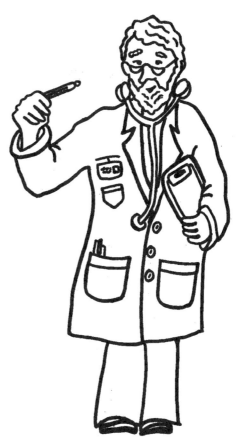

THE SCRIPT

A doctor's waiting room. A very efficient Nurse Able enters.

NURSE: Welcome to Doctor Bumblebee's surgery everyone. I am Nurse Able. The doctor will be with us shortly, but before he arrives, I need to take down some particulars from all of you.

Nurse Able goes up to each participant and starts to fill in the medical checklist.

> **NOTE:** If it is a large group and filling out a form for each participant would be too time-consuming, direct the questions to the whole group, filling in one form for all of them.

NURSE: Hello. What is your name?

She writes this down.

NURSE: Right [name], have you ever been sick before? Have you ever had a cough?

She demonstrates a cough.

NURSE: Have you ever had a sneeze?

She demonstrates a sneeze and so forth, encouraging the participants to demonstrate as well.

NURSE: Can you show me?

Once the medical checklist is completed, Nurse Able introduces Doctor Bumblebee.

NURSE: Well, I seem to have all of the details I need, so let me go and see if Doctor Bumblebee is ready for you now.

Nurse Able leaves as we hear her calling.

NURSE: Doctor, the patients are ready.

Nurse Able re-enters with Doctor Bumblebee.

Routledge
Taylor & Francis Group

DOCTOR: Well hello everybody. I'm Doctor Bumblebee. It's very good to see you all. Now where's your chart?

Nurse Able passes Doctor Bumblebee the group's medical checklist.

NURSE: Here you are Doctor.

DOCTOR: Now let me see. Dear oh dear. This doesn't look good. I think we'll have to operate. Now who would like to be the patient?

Nurse Able sets up both the operating table (with the sheet over it) and hangs up the 'Vital Organs of the Body' chart. Doctor Bumblebee casts the patient from the group and gets them to lie down on the table with the box of props (picture representations of the vital organs and some silly objects) underneath.

DOCTOR: Alrighty, let's see what we've got here.

He reaches into the box of props.

DOCTOR: Look what I've found, a [item]!

NURSE: What's that doing in there?

DOCTOR: I don't know.

This page may be photocopied for instructional use only. Drama Scripts for People with Special Needs © Sheree Vickers 2005

Routledge
Taylor & Francis Group

To the patient and the group.

DOCTOR: Do you need it?

PATIENT: Yes or No?

DOCTOR: Check the chart. Check the chart. Is the object on there? No. Let's try again.

Doctor Bumblebee gives the object to Nurse Able, who throws it away or places it in a box marked 'No'. If the object pulled out is a vital organ and the patient or group replies 'No', check the chart and guide them into the appropriate answer.

DOCTOR: Look the [heart]!

NURSE: What's that doing in there?

DOCTOR: I don't know.

To patient

DOCTOR: Do you need it?

PATIENT: Yes or No!

DOCTOR: Check the chart. Check the chart. Is the vital organ on there?

Go through the organs until you find a match and stick the picture onto the chart.

DOCTOR: Yes. It is on there. Wonderful! Let's see what else we have in here.

Doctor Bumblebee then pulls another strange object out of the patient's stomach and the process continues until all of the vital organs have been found.

DOCTOR: I think we've finished. Have we found all the vital organs? Let's check.

Run through the vital organs chart one more time.

DOCTOR: Alrighty, let's see the medical checklist again.

Nurse Able hands over the group's medical checklist. Doctor speaks aloud as writing on the chart.

DOCTOR: 'Clean bill of health. Signed, Doctor Bumblebee.' Here you are Nurse Able. I'm off to play a round of golf. Goodbye everyone.

Doctor Bumblebee exits as Nurse Able finishes the drama.

NURSE: Congratulations everyone. Your medical checklist is completely fine. Thank you all for helping us to find the vital organs, and remember, stay healthy.

Nurse Able packs away the operating table and exits.

Routledge
Taylor & Francis Group

Further ideas for a sensory workshop

- A texture, prop or sound can accompany each initial ailment that Nurse Able ticks off on the medical checklist. For example, in Flour Sneeze (see the Explanation of Activities chapter), bubbles for the coughing and a penny-whistle slide sound for falling down.

- Pass around each silly prop pulled out of the patient for the group to explore, reiterating that a 'teddy bear' doesn't belong inside a patient's stomach. Alternatively, to explore texture further, contrast soft and hard props (such as small beanbags and stones), telling the group that the soft props are the ones needed and the hard ones should be left out.

- Dress the group up as doctors and nurses.

Additional games and activities

- Combine with the 'Training Day' script and train the group up as doctors and nurses etc.

- Extend the question on the medical checklist to do with falling down, by using bandages to wrap up the group and helping them to identify various parts of the body, for example, putting the arm in a sling or bandaging the foot.

Alternative scenarios for future dramas

Travelling the world

The group wants to go on holiday and needs to pack a suitcase for that particular country. They could be in a travel agent's shop or at an airport.

Replace the character of Nurse Able with a travel agent, the doctor with a holiday-maker and the patient could be a person holding the suitcase, for example 'Now let me see. Dear oh dear. This doesn't look good. I think we'll have to repack. Now who would like to help me hold the suitcase?'

Checklist questions could include, 'Have you ever been on holiday before?', 'Where did you go?', 'How did you get there?' (aeroplane, bus, car etc).

The wall chart should contain all the essentials for travelling to that particular location, for example, if in a hot country, suntan lotion, or if camping, a tent.

Routledge
Taylor & Francis Group

The chef's kitchen

The group is visiting the school kitchen to learn how to eat a healthy lunch.

Replace Nurse Able with a dinner lady, Doctor Bumblebee with a chef and the patients can be holding the lunch box or picnic hamper.

Checklist questions could include 'Have you ever made your own lunch before?', 'Do you have any food allergies?', 'What are your favourite foods?'

You could finish the session with the group actually cooking and preparing a meal.

Appropriate behaviour

The group is visiting a school playground to learn how to behave towards others.

Replace Nurse Able with the school secretary, Doctor Bumblebee with the head teacher and the patient could be a character who is hoping to join the group and wants to make friends.

Checklist questions could include 'Have you ever felt scared?', 'Do you like playing games?', 'Who are your friends?' etc.

The wall chart could contain good words and behaviour pictures such as 'sharing', 'please' or pictures of someone asking for help and smiling, with inappropriate words put into the 'No' box.

This time in history

Visit any time in history and replace the characters accordingly. For example, would a peasant in medieval times have a microwave oven, or would George Washington have travelled around on a motorbike? This scenario can also be adapted to explore geography and to discover what is appropriate for each country or continent, such as camels in the Sahara and kangaroos in Australia.

Routledge
Taylor & Francis Group

Medical Checklist

NAME

Have you had any of the following?

Cough ☐

Sneeze ☐

Fallen down ☐

Use the check boxes below to note how your fall was treated.

Sticky plaster ☐   Stitches ☐

Plaster cast ☐   Kiss ☐

Sore throat ☐

Had your temperature taken? ☐

Had an injection? ☐

Had your heart listened to? ☐

Any additional information

Signed by Doctor Bumblebee:

Routledge
Taylor & Francis Group

ROUTLEDGE

PROFESSOR WAFFLEPUFF

This basic format is ideal for teaching not only the importance of rules, but also a variety of science topics.

NOTE: It is always a good idea to practise the experiments before the drama session to establish which quantities work best.

Props List

- Professor Wafflepuff's ID badge (already pinned on to coat)
- ID badges (see p36)
- Food colourings (red, yellow, blue and green)
- Bicarbonate of soda
- Vinegar
- Clear plastic cups
- White coat
- Two specimen bottles, both marked 'Caution. Be careful!', one containing vinegar, the other bicarbonate of soda (both placed in coat pocket)
- Botchy's costume or hat
- A list of the rules (placed in coat pocket) (see p36)
- A bottle of water or access to running water
- A pair of prop reading glasses (optional)
- Celebration music and a CD or tape player
- A jellybean or other edible type 'pill'
- A feather duster (optional)

Character List

Professor Wafflepuff

Assistant Botchy

Visitors (or Trainee Scientists)

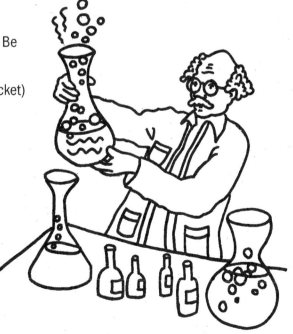

THE SCRIPT

A table with the necessary scientific equipment is set up at the back of the room. Enter and address the group as yourself.

> **NOTE:** This opening introduction into Professor Wafflepuff's character can be skipped or shortened if the group is comfortable with role play or this particular format.

You: Look what I've found everybody.

Hold up the white coat.

You: What do you think it is? Who do you think it belongs to?

Take suggestions.

You: It could be, but look, it's got a name badge on it.

Read the name badge.

You: 'Professor Wafflepuff – scientist'. This coat belongs to Professor Wafflepuff, who is a scientist. Who knows what a scientist is? What sort of things do they do?

Take suggestions and guide the participants to the correct answers.

You: Look what else I've found. I wonder what they are?

Take out the bicarbonate of soda and vinegar specimen jars. As they are clearly labelled 'Caution. Be careful!', show them to the group, reading the labels and discussing what they mean before replacing them in the coat pocket and discovering the list of rules.

You: And look what else I've found, a list of rules:
  1 *Be quiet when the experiments are in progress.*
  2 *Don't touch anything unless asked.*
  3 *Always clean up.*

Read, repeat and discuss the list of rules before replacing them in the coat pocket.

You: Would you like to meet Professor Wafflepuff and see what she is doing?

> **NOTE:** If the group answers 'No' to meeting Professor Wafflepuff, and appears quite nervous at the prospect, find a pair of dummy reading glasses in the pocket of the coat and use them to gain the group's sympathy. For example 'She can't see without her glasses. Who thinks they're brave enough or kind enough to give her back her glasses?' Give the glasses to that person, put the coat on and begin as Professor Wafflepuff by asking the participants if they have seen her glasses. Put them on and proceed with the drama. Alternatively, see the 'Dragon Sleep' script for a step-by-step breakdown on introducing a character.

Put on the white coat and address the group.

WAFFLEPUFF: Greetings everyone. Welcome to my laboratory. Do you have your ID badges on? You don't? Well, I can't let you into the laboratory without your ID badges. Now let me see, where did I put them? Oh, here they are. Right, what's your name?

Go up to each participant, write their name down and give them a badge. Alternatively, hand out existing badges made in a previous session (see 'Additional Games and Activities' at the end of this script).

WAFFLEPUFF: Now that we all have our name badges on, let me start again. Greetings everyone. Welcome to my laboratory. There are three rules that must be obeyed in this laboratory. Do you know what those three rules are?

If needed, bring out the list of rules from the coat pocket to prompt the group. Alternatively, hang up the list of rules for people to see.

WAFFLEPUFF: That's right, Number one: 'Be quiet' – especially when I'm mixing up my potions. Number two: 'Don't touch anything' – this is very important because there can be some very dangerous things in a laboratory.

> **NOTE:** The group may raise questions about the vials labelled 'Caution. Be careful!' at this point. If so, take them out of your pocket with a comment such as, 'Thanks for reminding me' and place them gently on one end of the table. If further questioning persists, elaborate by mentioning how they are two very smelly potions that should never be mixed.

WAFFLEPUFF: And Number three: 'Always clean up' – do you ever have to clean up stuff? What sorts of things do you clean up?

Take or prompt suggestions.

WAFFLEPUFF: I wish I had you all to help me instead of my assistant Botchy. Have you met Botchy yet? You haven't! He's hopeless. He keeps getting everything wrong and he's very lazy. He always wears a [hat].

Show the group Botchy's costume or hat.

WAFFLEPUFF: Keep an eye out for him. Anyway, would you like to help me today? I'm busy making colours.

Take the group to the preset table and seat them in a formation where they can all see the experiments. Explain the layout of the table to the group.

> **NOTE:** If guiding someone else in role, cast yourself as a good assistant (keeping someone else as Botchy, the naughty assistant) guiding with questions such as 'What experiments are you doing today?', 'What equipment do we have here?', etc.

WAFFLEPUFF: I have here four cups of water.

In clear cups for the group to see the contents.

WAFFLEPUFF: I am trying to make four colours – red, yellow, green and blue. I have been trying for such a long time, but I think today I might just be able to do it. If I do succeed in making the colours, I will finally be able to celebrate. I've been wanting to celebrate for such a long time now. Do you know how I celebrate? I dance. I put this music on and dance to it.

Put the celebration music on and demonstrate Professor Wafflepuff's dancing. Encourage the group to join in before abruptly switching the music off.

WAFFLEPUFF: But we can't celebrate until I've succeeded in my experiments.

> **NOTE:** If the group is unaccustomed to certain scientific terms, explain the dialogue with a follow-up line. Taking the line above as an example, say the line as written and then immediately follow with, 'So we can't dance until I've made the colours.' This defines the meaning of new words and repeats the instructions. For a further example on repeating and clarifying dialogue, see the 'Macbeth' workshop breakdown, which constantly defines Shakespeare's text.

WAFFLEPUFF: Are we ready? I'm going to try and make [blue].

Pick up one of the food colourings and a clear cup of water.

WAFFLEPUFF: Remember, we need to be very, very quiet.

Very slowly and with great importance, drop some food colouring into the clear water. Allow it to mix and hold it up for the group to see.

> **NOTE:** The aim is to get the group focused on the experiment, so use your discretion if total silence is impossible to achieve. Despite the note on not acting in the 'Introduction', the success of the group's focus relies on your commitment to the experiment. Therefore, if you believe this is the most important experiment in the world, the group will believe it too.

WAFFLEPUFF: What colour do I have? [blue] I've succeeded! We've made blue! Let's dance.

Enjoy a short celebratory dance before abruptly switching the music off and continuing.

WAFFLEPUFF: We can't celebrate forever. I still have three colours to make. This time, I'm going to make [yellow].

Pick up the next food colouring and another clear cup of water. Repeat the experiment and celebration dance process until all four colours have been made.

WAFFLEPUFF: Congratulations everyone. We've made the colours red, green, blue and yellow. We've celebrated with our dancing and now, let me just check my rules. Yes! It's time to clean up. I don't know where my assistant Botchy is, so I'm afraid I'm going to need your help with this.

If it hasn't happened already, remove the bicarbonate of soda and vinegar specimen bottles from the coat pocket and gently place them on the table before playing the 'Clean-up' mime game (see the Explanation of Activities chapter). Once the specific clean-up activities are established, Professor Wafflepuff disappears and assistant Botchy enters.

WAFFLEPUFF: Keep cleaning everyone. I'm going to see where my lazy assistant Botchy is.

Botchy enters and promptly falls asleep in the middle of the room, snoring and grumpy.

BOTCHY: Auurrghh. What's all this noise? I'm trying to sleep.

This page may be photocopied for instructional use only. *Drama Scripts for People with Special Needs* © Sheree Vickers 2005

Routledge
Taylor & Francis Group

BOTCHY: I don't want to do any cleaning. I'm too tired. Auurrghh. What are you waking me up for? What's all this you're doing?

Get each specific cleaning task from the group.

BOTCHY: You're [sweeping]? How do you [sweep]? Is it like this?

Start sweeping and then promptly fall asleep again, ready for the group to wake you up. Repeat this reluctant cleaning/sleeping activity for as long as appropriate, even asking members of the group if they would like to be the sleeping Botchy.

BOTCHY: Alright everyone. I get the message. Auurrghh. I'll keep cleaning up. You can all go and sit back down now. I promise I'll clean.

Get the group sitting down before discovering the experiments table.

BOTCHY: Auurrghh. What's this? Oh yeah, Professor Wafflepuff's experiments table. She's been trying to make colours. She should have asked me. I know how to make colours ...

Botchy picks up the vials of vinegar and bicarbonate of soda (both marked 'Caution. Be careful!') and proceeds to mix them together, which should create a wonderfully fizzy, albeit smelly, mixture.

BOTCHY: Auurrghh. Oh no. Professor Wafflepuff's not going to like this. I'm outta here. Bye.

Botchy makes a hasty exit. Professor Wafflepuff suddenly appears.

WAFFLEPUFF: My goodness. What happened here?

Responses from the group.

WAFFLEPUFF: Did my assistant Botchy do this? I don't know what I'm going to do with him. Do you have any ideas?

Take some suggestions.

WAFFLEPUFF: Those are all very good suggestions, but I think I know what to do.

Professor Wafflepuff produces a pill from her pocket.

WAFFLEPUFF: I have here a magic pill that, when taken, will turn Botchy into the best, most efficient assistant ever. Unfortunately it only works for a small amount of time, but it should be just enough time to get him to clean up this mess.

> **NOTE:** This version has been written to accommodate working solo. Alternatively, call the character of Botchy in and give him the pill yourself to continue with the drama.

WAFFLEPUFF: I'll just place it here. Make sure nobody but Botchy eats it.

Professor Wafflepuff exits. Botchy enters.

BOTCHY: Is the coast clear? Auurrghh. Good. I didn't want to have to clean up the mess ... Hello! What do we have here?

Botchy picks up the 'pill'.

BOTCHY: Yum!

As soon as Botchy eats the pill he becomes a very efficient cleaning machine.

BOTCHY: Oh no! Look at all this mess. Dear oh dear oh dear. We can't have this.

Botchy quickly repeats all the 'Clean-up' mime activities and packs away the experiments table. He could even pull out a feather duster and clean the participants.

BOTCHY: I certainly hope you didn't make this mess.

Repeat to individuals, using their names.

Routledge
Taylor & Francis Group

BOTCHY: Look at this. It's dreadful.

When the cleaning has been done, Botchy starts to yawn.

BOTCHY: Auurrghh. I'm awfully tired again now. I think ... I'll go and lie down ... nighty night.

Botchy exits and Professor Wafflepuff re-enters.

WAFFLEPUFF: Just the way I like it. Did Botchy clean up everyone? I thought so. He's having a nice little nap now. Thank you for all your help. Please come and visit me in my laboratory again. Now that I've made my colours, I need to think up some new experiments. Goodbye everyone.

Professor Wafflepuff exits.

Routledge
Taylor & Francis Group

Further ideas for a sensory workshop

◌ Before discovering the list of rules, find a box of 'scientific props' for the group to explore. These could be general items (such as a magnifying glass, a battery or a magnet) or those more specific to the experiment (such as the clear plastic cups, water and vials).

◌ Replace the food-colouring experiment with a torch and some coloured scarves or cellophane. Cover the torchlight with the different coloured scarves or cellophane, dim the lights and change the colour of the room.

◌ Repeat Botchy's bicarbonate of soda and vinegar experiment personally for each participant. Break the process down by smelling the vinegar and feeling the bicarbonate, before mixing the two together.

◌ Change the lighting in the room for Botchy's entrance and experiment.

Additional games and activities

◌ Each participant can create their own ID badge, even drawing a small picture of himself.

◌ Use the food colouring water to paint onto a paper towel. When dry, the colours are visible. Play around with other watercolour painting effects, including running water over designs drawn with marker pens to watch the ink run, or over designs drawn with wax crayons to watch how the watercolours are not absorbed into the waxed areas.

◌ The group could make its own set of rules for different situations, for example crossing the street, entering the classroom, etc.

◌ With paint, try mixing prime colours to make other colours, such as yellow and red for orange, yellow and blue for green, and blue and red for purple.

◌ If the participants had a magic pill, what power would it allow them to have?

Alternative scenarios for future dramas

Use the same rules, characters and activities, but substitute the scientific experiments.

In the kitchen

Replace the laboratory with a kitchen in which Chef Terramina is trying to create a gourmet lunch. Botchy meanwhile brings in all the wrong ingredients, uses all the appliances badly (such as trying to cut bread with a fork), and he creates a large mess when his experiment (juggling with real eggs) goes wrong.

Routledge
Taylor & Francis Group

The artist's workshop

The famous artist Madam Poffle is creating some amazing pieces of artwork with different paint effects (or modelling figures with clay, or, if you have access to a washing machine, try some tie-dying). Botchy makes a mess by mixing all the paints wrong and turning Madam's colour palette into a yucky brown colour.

Cleaning nonsense

Cleaning lady Betsy is keeping the room looking spick and span. Botchy, however, uses the vacuum cleaner to clean the windows, the kitchen cloth to clean the carpets and the curtains to clean the toilet.

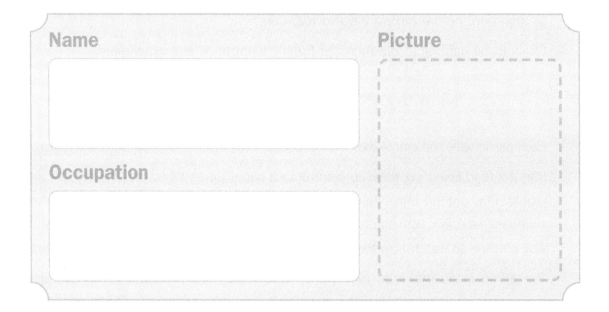

Name

Picture

Occupation

Laboratory Rules

1. BE QUIET when the experiments are in progress

2. DON'T TOUCH ANYTHING unless asked

3. ALWAYS CLEAN UP

DRAGON SLEEP

In this script, the group encounters a dragon, which must be defeated and befriended. The group will learn about bullying, overcoming fear and forging friendships.

NOTE: The tactics used for defeating the dragon are never violent. Any reference to killing the creature or tying it up and hurting it in anyway are gently discouraged with phrases such as, 'That's one idea, but we need to try this first. If it doesn't work, then we'll go to Plan B'.

Character List

The King (or Queen)

Knights

Princesses

Wizard Spinkin

A Dragon

Props List

▪ A crown for the King (or Queen)

▪ A wizard's hat or cape

▪ Material for the dragon

▪ Knights' and princesses' props, such as wands, crowns, shields and (optional) swords

▪ A treasure of gold coins and jewels

NOTE: These props can be imagined if the group is able to pretend, alternatively they can be made in a preliminary session or during the drama, as preparation for the quest.

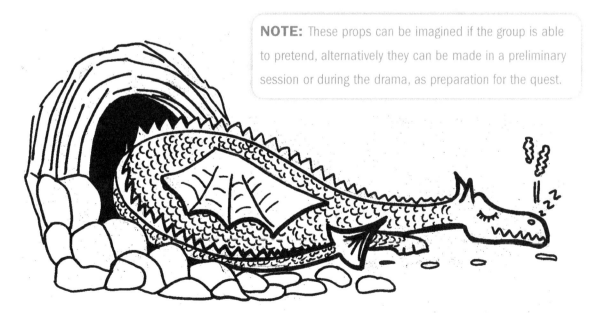

THE SCRIPT

KING: Welcome, loyal subjects. I am the king of this land and I need your help. There is a ferocious dragon who lives in a cave at the top of a mountain. He has taken all our gold and jewels, and I need some very brave knights and princesses to go and get them back. Can you all show me your brave faces?

Use names, demonstrate and repeat as necessary.

KING: Can you show me your scared faces? That's wonderful. I'm pretty scared myself. Show me your brave faces again. Wonderful! So who would like to go on this quest to see the dragon and rescue the treasure?

> **NOTE:** If a great majority of the group don't wish to go, or are too frightened by the concept, confirm that it is OK to be scared and allow them to watch the drama from the sidelines. Continue to include them from their safe place, always giving them the option of joining in the drama at any point. Also reiterate that they don't have to meet the dragon if they don't want to. If necessary, drop role to remind them that this is pretend.

Allow the group to choose their roles as either knights or princesses.

KING: Welcome [name], are you going to be a knight or a princess?

Give each participant either a crown and wand or a shield and sword, depending on who they wish to be. Once everyone is ready, ask them to sit down.

KING: You all look marvellous. Now there is one very special person who can tell us more about the dragon and how to get our treasure back. Let me introduce you to Wizard Spinkin.

> **NOTE:** If casting Wizard Spinkin from the group, guide the dialogue as the King with questions such as, 'How do we put the dragon to sleep?', 'Are there any magic words?', and so forth.

Wizard Spinkin enters.

WIZARD: Hello, hello, hello. So you're off to meet the dragon. Well, well, well. I know what you must do. The dragon roars like this ...

Either demonstrate the dragon's roar or get the group to decide on a roar, for example 'Do you know how the dragon roars?', 'Can you show me?'

WIZARD: Can you all show me your roars? Lovely, lovely, lovely. Now in order to get the treasure back you must put the dragon to sleep. Do you know how to put the dragon to sleep?

Adapt the following dialogue to give the participants the opportunity to decide on the magic words and/or actions themselves.

WIZARD: Correct, correct, correct. There are magic words and they are 'booley shoosh booley shoosh waa waa waa'.

Add (or develop with the group) actions to go with the magic words.

WIZARD: Can you all do that with me?

Repeat and practise the magic words with the actions.

WIZARD: Yes, yes, yes. You are now ready to face the dragon.

KING: Show me your brave faces once more everyone.

Encourage the group to do so.

KING: Good luck and I'll see you when you return.

Drop the role by removing the king and/or wizard costume and address the group as yourself.

NOTE: The following breakdown can be shortened or skipped entirely if the group is comfortable with role play or this particular format. It is used to help those scared by the idea of a dragon, breaking down its creation and empowering the participants with the job of developing its character. It is also a beneficial sequence for demonstrating the dragon role before casting somebody else. (If an individual from the group is taking on the role, allow for spontaneous dialogue that could even affect the reason the dragon stole the treasure in the first place.)

You: I am now going to become the dragon. This material is going to be used for the dragon character, but I'm not sure how to wear it. Should I wear it like this?

Put the material over your head.

You: How about like this?

Put the material around your waist.

You: Or how about this?

Put the material as a cape around your neck.

You: I think I'll wear it like this. What do you think?

Generally the group will decide how it wants the material to be worn. Encourage the participants further by asking for a volunteer to come up and help dress you.

You: Now, what type of roar do you think the dragon might have?

Elicit ideas and practise their suggestions.

You: Do you think he might sound like this?

Roar 1.

You: How about this?

Roar 2.

You: Would it be loud or soft?

Demonstrate.

You: What about movement? Would his body be tall [stretch up tall], or short? [Crouch down low.]

Recap the group's dragon character suggestions.

You: So I'm wearing my costume like this ...

Put the material on.

You: ... and I'm roaring like this ...

Demonstrate roar.

You: ... and I'm moving like this ...

Show the group tall or small.

YOU: Alright, let me practise.

Practise the group's suggestions, even getting them wrong a couple of times.

YOU: How was that? Did I do it right? Excellent. Are you all ready to meet the dragon then?

Go into role as the dragon, carrying some of the gold coins and jewellery, and roaring.

DRAGON: Well, hello. Why are you all here? Are you trying to get this lovely treasure back? Well there's no way anyone can get this treasure. It's mine and I'm keeping it. Unless you know the magic words for putting me to sleep? Does anyone know the magic words for putting me to sleep? I hope not.

> **NOTE:** A good helper is essential at this point to help guide and encourage the participants. If you are working alone however, drop role and demonstrate to the knights and princesses exactly what is going to happen next.

Drop role and address the group.

YOU: Do you remember the magic words everyone? What are they?

Remind the group and practise.

YOU: Excellent! This is what's going to happen ...

Demonstrate as you speak.

YOU: On your own or with a partner, you are going to sneak up to the dragon and when he asks you what you want, you are going to say the magic words, 'booley shoosh booley shoosh waa waa waa'. The dragon will then fall asleep and you can steal the treasure back. So who would like to come up first?

> **NOTE:** Occasionally there is an absolute refusal to sneak up to the dragon. Should this happen, put the dragon's costume on the floor covering the treasure. Re-join the group and sneak up quietly to the 'sleeping dragon'. Lift the costume, find the treasure and run back to the group. Replace the treasure and repeat this hide-and-seek adaptation with individual participants.

Place the volunteers in the space; practise with them again if necessary before going back into role as the dragon.

DRAGON: So you think you know the magic words do you? Let me hear them?

Encourage the group to say the magic words. Become drowsy as the dragon, yawn, stretch and lie down snoring (always keeping one eye on the group). The volunteer knights and/or princesses should then take the treasure and run back to their places.

> **NOTE:** If the group has not taken the initiative to steal back the treasure while the dragon is sleeping, drop hints, such as 'Nothing like a good nap. I hope they don't take my jewels', etc.

The dragon wakes up.

DRAGON: Huh! Huh? Where's my treasure? Who stole my treasure? Never mind. It's a good thing I've got some more.

The dragon goes and gets some more treasure, and roars.

DRAGON: You won't get this lovely treasure back. It's mine and I'm keeping it. Unless you know the magic words for putting me to sleep? I hope not.

Repeat the process of sneaking up on the dragon and retrieving the treasure. Continue with the script until all the treasure has been retrieved.

DRAGON: All of my lovely treasure is gone. All gone. Do you know why I stole it? I just wanted some company. No one ever comes to see me. I have no friends.

The dragon sits down and starts to cry.

DRAGON: Everyone's afraid of me. I don't mean to scare people, but I don't know what to do.

Drop role and address the group.

YOU: Oh dear everyone. What should we do about the dragon? He's not very happy is he? Do you think he's very mean and scary after all? What was it that he wanted? Do you think maybe that we could help him get some friends? What sort of things does a good friend do?

Take suggestions, compile a list and ask some members of the group to present the list to the dragon. (Either take the role back on yourself, or ask if someone else would like to be the dragon.)

Routledge
Taylor & Francis Group

> **NOTE:** Sometimes a suggestion is made to give the treasure back. Your response could be in the positive, such as 'What a nice idea', but then, when back in role as the dragon, tell them that, as you'd stolen it in the first place and you now realise that stealing was wrong, they had better keep the treasure and return it to its rightful owner.

DRAGON: [Who is still sitting and sobbing.] I've got no friends. Waaaa. I don't know what to do.

The dragon notices the people approaching him with a list.

DRAGON: What's this? It's a list. What does it say?

He reads the list.

DRAGON: You made this list for me? That's the nicest thing anyone has ever done for me. Waaaa. [He starts crying again.] Thank you all very much. Waaaa. I'm just going to go back into my cave and blow my nose. Waaaa. Promise me you'll all come again and visit soon. Do you promise? Waaaa. That's so nice. Waaaa. I'll see you soon. Bye.

The dragon exits.

YOU: We'd better get back to the King everyone. Do you have the treasure? Great. Let's sing a song on the way back.

Sing to the tune of 'The Bear Went Over The Mountain'.

ALL: *We went to visit a dragon*
We went to visit a dragon
We went to visit a dragon to get our treasure back.
And all that we could see
And all that we could see
Was a very lonely dragon
A very lonely dragon
A very lonely dragon was all that we could see.

By the end of the song, the king has reappeared.

KING: Welcome back loyal subjects. Did you retrieve the treasure? Wonderful! And how was the dragon? Was he scary?

Prompt the group into re-telling their adventure, including befriending the dragon.

This page may be photocopied for instructional use only. Drama Scripts for People with Special Needs © Sheree Vickers 2005

KING: So he wasn't scary? He just wanted some friends? Well, I'm so glad you managed to teach him all about that. And now, my loyal subjects, for returning the treasure to the kingdom, we are going to hold a royal dance.

End with a formal dance where the knights and princesses play musical chairs (see 'Musical Statues Sshoosh' in the Explanation of Activities chapter).

Routledge
Taylor & Francis Group

Further ideas for a sensory workshop

- Have a special effect for Wizard Spinkin's entrance, for example a specific piece of music, or get the group to summon him with musical instruments (see 'Sound Orchestra' in the Explanation of Activities chapter).

- Create a dragon's lair full of different textures. Turn the lights out and put on some mood music. Egg boxes provide a wonderful texture. Hang them from the ceiling for the group to move through, or tape them to a wall for a large dragon skin collage.

- Do a 'Parachute Run' (see the Explanation of Activities chapter) away from the dragon.

- Replace the list of things a good friend does with actions, for example giving the dragon a gentle touch (just as when stroking a cat) and speaking softly to people, as opposed to a loud noise or yelling. Other suggested actions could be a hug, a kiss on the hand, or a smile.

- The dragon might scare everyone away with 'Balloon Water Bombs' (see 'Balloon Tricks' in the Explanation of Activities chapter).

Additional games and activities

- Ask each participant to come up with a letter-match name for their knight or princess, for example Stuart the Scary or Bernadette the Beautiful.

- End with a ceremony where the King proudly presents the group with medals of bravery and friendship.

- Extend the dragon quest with a longer journey, possibly across a river (create a hopscotch design for the group to jump across as stepping stones), through a forest (create some forest sounds, make some trees, camp for the night around a fire and tell some stories or sing some songs), up a mountain and through a cave – the group may even wish to take a train.

- Use the 'Training Day' script to train the group as knights and princesses, learning skills such as bowing and curtseys, royal waving, jousting, riding horses and kissing frogs!

Routledge
Taylor & Francis Group

Alternative scenarios for future dramas

Changes to the ending

- Instead of becoming friends, the dragon might need to learn to share. Therefore, replace the gold and jewels with food that has been stolen from a starving kingdom.

- The dragon might smell and need to learn to bathe properly.

- The dragon has no friends because he doesn't know how to use the bus and can't visit anyone.

The haunted house

(As in the 'My Neighbourhood' script.)

Replace the dragon with a ghost, Wizard Spinkin with a fortune-teller and the king with the house's owner who is too scared to investigate and has hired professional help in this team of brave ghost catchers.

Running away from the dog

From the 'Training Day' script, where a noisy dog is preventing the Postman from delivering mail to this address.

The storm monster

A dreadful storm is coming and the only way to stop it is to visit the Storm Monster. He creates a dreadful racket with his instruments (which need to be taken away) and can only be tamed by giggling (which is infectious and makes him laugh also).

This is a lovely concept with which to explore weather conditions and what causes them, possibly even meeting other elemental creatures along the way, such as Windy Wally and Sunny Sagerine.

Routledge
Taylor & Francis Group

MY NEIGHBOURHOOD

The purpose of this script is to meet different people and encounter different situations while on a mission to return a lost item to its rightful owner.

It can be adapted to create any form of journey.

First worked with small groups of 16–20-year-old students with mixed abilities, from Down's syndrome to severe and complex learning difficulties, for POLKA Theatre's 2004 production of 'Hey There Boy With The BeBop'.

Props List

- A tape with Elvis Presley's 'Hound Dog' on it (and marked 'Property of Rockin' Rudolf. Please Return.')
- A wig and scarf for Mama's character
- Various hats, scarves, wigs, material and dressing-up costumes to help match the chosen characters of the neighbourhood
- Different types of music (including another copy of 'Hound Dog') and a CD or tape player

Character List

- Narrator
- Mama (a nosey old lady)
- Various characters from the neighbourhood

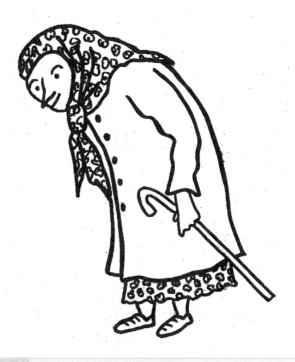

THE SCRIPT

NARRATOR: We are going to dress up and do some acting. What sort of character do you think might wear this type of hat?

Bring out the collection of hats, scarves, wigs, material and dressing-up costumes to explore. For example, a woollen hat could be introduced by asking 'Would you wear this type of hat if it was hot or cold?' Put the hat on and shiver as though it were very cold. Pass the hat around for others to try on and shiver. Repeat the exploration with two or three other hats before discovering Mama's wig and scarf.

NARRATOR: So if I put this wig and scarf on, what sort of character do you think I might be?

Put on the wig and scarf and become Mama.

MAMA: Oooh, hello everyone. What are you doing in my neighbourhood? What's your name? Oooh, aren't you lovely! Welcome to my neighbourhood. I've lived here all my life.

> **NOTE:** The character of Mama has produced some startling reactions in the group, from being very protective, to wishing she would go away. She is wonderful to improvise with, but should the character start to impede the drama, or you don't feel comfortable with her (or him), return to the more neutral role of Narrator.

MAMA: I found this tape. [name] is it yours? It's got 'Property of Rockin' Rudolf. Please Return' written on it. You're not Rockin' Rudolf!

Repeat to various participants. Usually they will prompt Mama into playing it, but if not, lead into it yourself.

MAMA: Shall we play it?

Play the tape and listen to the opening section of 'Hound Dog', then switch off the tape recorder and take the tape out of the player.

MAMA: Oooh, it's a bit loud.

Routledge
Taylor & Francis Group

Reading the tape again.

MAMA: 'Property of Rockin' Rudolf. Please Return.' What shall we do with it? [name] what shall we do with it? It has 'Property of Rockin' Rudolf. Please Return', written on it.

Mama is usually prompted into returning the tape as well.

MAMA: Shall we return it? Well, I can't quite remember which door it is. Let's go and have a look. Are you going to come with me?

If possible, get the group to line up and follow the leader as the rhyme is said. Otherwise, get Mama walking around the participants, ready to choose the first character.

MAMA: There's a little rhyme I like to say as we go. It goes like this ...
I wonder who lives here?
I wonder who lives there?
We seem to be quite near.
Let's knock upon the door ... Knock ... Knock ... Knock

The group starts to knock (either on an actual door or by saying 'Knock, Knock, Knock' as they do the actions). While they're knocking a piece of music is played.

MAMA: Oooh, everybody. Listen.

Mama has an appropriate reaction to each different piece of music and helps to guide the participants back to their places. For example, with haunted house spooky music, she gets scared and shuffles everyone quickly back to their seats. With the heavy metal punk music, she puts her fingers in her ears before getting them all to sit down.

MAMA: Does it match the music on the tape?

Listen and compare if necessary.

MAMA: It doesn't does it? Who do you think lives here?

Take suggestions.

MAMA: Oooh, I remember who lives here ...

See Table 1 for different characters and music suggestions.

Musical suggestions

MUSIC SUGGESTION	CHARACTER	ACTIVITY
Traditional Chinese	Karate expert	Karate Chop Duck Game
Spooky music	Ghost in a haunted house	Run Away Boo!
Heavy metal	Punk	Musical Statues Sshoosh
Tchaikovsky's The Nutcracker	A ballerina (as a group or individually)	Dance around on tiptoes
Gershwin's Rhapsody in Blue	A burglar and police officer	Who's Got the Jewels? or Grandmother's Footsteps
Calliope music	A clown	Pull silly faces

Turn the music off, take off Mama's wig and scarf and return to the role of Narrator.

NARRATOR: Who would like to be [character name]? What sort of thing do you think he might wear?

NOTE: Generally in a one-hour session, introducing the group to two or three different characters is ample before discovering Rockin' Rudolf's house. Table 1 offers suggestions for characters, music and activities to choose from.

Decide on a costume and prepare for each activity (see the Explanation of Activities chapter for a breakdown of certain games).

NARRATOR: Hello [name]. What sort of music are you listening to? I know about that sort of music. Can we all join you in ... ? Do you know how to play it? Well, it goes like this.

Once the activity is over, address the character directly.

NARRATOR: That was so much fun, but we're looking for Rockin' Rudolf. He's lost his tape. Do you know him?

It doesn't matter what the answer is, but if the answer is 'Yes', ask for directions before the group moves on to another house.

Routledge
Taylor & Francis Group

NARRATOR: Thank you for letting us visit. Bye.

Give the person playing that particular character a round of applause, getting them to return their costume and reintroducing Mama, who is wearing the wig and scarf again.

MAMA: Oooh, hello everyone. Did you find Rockin' Rudolf? Did you return his tape? No? What were you doing in that house all that time? Who did you meet? What were you doing?

Guide the group into recapping the activities so far.

MAMA: We still haven't found Rockin' Rudolf. We'll have to knock on another door. OK, everybody get ready.

Say the 'I Wonder Who Lives Here' follow-the-leader rhyme again and meet another character. When enough characters have been met for the session, discover Rockin' Rudolf by playing Elvis Presley's 'Hound Dog' while the group is busy knocking.

MAMA: Oooh, everybody. Listen. Does it match the music on the tape? It does! We've found him!

Turn the music off. Get the participants to return to their places and cast Rockin' Rudolf in the same manner as the others.

NARRATOR: Who would like to be Rockin' Rudolf? What sort of thing do you think he might wear?

Choose a costume and dress character before returning to the role of Mama.

MAMA: Rockin' Rudolf, we have something of yours.

To the group.

MAMA: Who would like to give the tape back to Rockin' Rudolf?

The tape is returned either by Mama or by a member of the group.

MAMA: Oooh, shall we play it? Will you teach me how to dance? Who would like to dance with us?

End the session with everyone dancing in the space or extend it by having a fun 1950's dress party.

Routledge
Taylor & Francis Group

Further ideas for a sensory workshop

Either take on the various neighbourhood characters yourself, interacting with each participant, or spend time dressing the group as the characters and showing them the transformation in a mirror. Use the following rhyme to help dress each character:

All sorts of people like to wear a hat.

Choose one. Try one.

How about ... that!

Suggested changes and additions to the various activities:

- Traditional Chinese – try some Chinese food, wave a Chinese fan in front of the participants' faces, or, if playing 'Karate Chop Duck', physically move their hands, bodies and/or wheelchairs.

- Spooky music – change the lighting in the room and brush a sheet across individuals in the group. Possibly do some trick-or-treating and eat the sweets collected.

- Heavy metal – dress the group up as punks using hair gel or wigs.

- Tchaikovsky's *The Nutcracker* – pass around a pair of ballerina's shoes or tutu material.

- Gershwin's *Rhapsody in Blue* – Pass around and hide a bag full of jewels. Play the burglar trying to find them.

- Calliope music – pull silly faces in front of the mirror and use face paint to dress as clowns.

Additional games and activities

- Draw a map of the neighbourhood and all the people who live in it.

- Play hopscotch, ball games and various other outdoor games (see 'Mime Freeze' activity in the Explanation of Activities chapter).

- Explore the theme of gossip and rumours by having Mama say outlandish things about Rockin' Rudolf, for example, 'He's got three heads and eats dinosaurs for tea'. The group's journey could also include convincing Mama that this gossip is untrue.

- Adapt the script by replacing Mama with a detective looking for clues. Every character the detective meets gives him a piece of the puzzle that helps to build the final character, for example, a shirt, a hat, the tape, etc.

Routledge
Taylor & Francis Group

◎ This script is also ideal for exploring the theme of other people's property and what it feels like to lose something precious. Each character along the way has lost something and it is the group's job to match the item to the character.

Alternative scenarios for future dramas

Inside the house

Knocking on sister's, mother's or brother's room and discovering either music, smells or items for each before finding your own room. Could also include other rooms, such as the kitchen, bathroom, garage, etc.

What job is that?

The group needs to return an item related to a specific occupation, for example a spoon or a hammer. (Change the words in the 'I Wonder Who Lives Here' follow-the-leader song to 'I Wonder Who Works Here?').

Suggested jobs and activities could include:

◎ A laundromat – with bubbles and the 'Wash Rinse Spin' game (see the Explanation of Activities chapter)

◎ A bakery – 'Flour Sneeze' (see the Explanation of Activities chapter): play with dough, cook and/or eat some bread and other bakery products

◎ The doctors – bandage the group up while naming parts of the body (extend with 'The Operation' script)

◎ A watchmaker – listen to the sound of different clocks

◎ School teacher – play an adaptation of 'Musical Statues Sshoosh' (see the Explanation of Activities chapter) where the group makes noise in a classroom

◎ The telephone exchange – a telephone rings with various conversations or questions for each participant.

Other professional characters could include a police officer, a cashier at the supermarket, or a movie star.

Fairy tales

'I found this red cape. It says "Property of Little Red Riding Hood. Please Return" on it.' Each door knocked upon reveals a different fairy tale, which could end by teaching Red Riding Hood how to escape from the wolf or sitting down to tea with Grandma.

Animals at the zoo

Each animal makes a different sound and has different textures, and it is the job of the group to return a special feather to its rightful owner. Add further drama by adding a time limit to the task. For example, 'If we don't return this feather in time, the dodo bird is in danger of extinction.' The location could change to a farm, a vet or a safari with animals specific to that location.

Different countries and nationalities

Explore recipes and different types of food from each location.

Shopping for wizard supplies

Originally worked to accompany the Harry Potter books, each shop contains necessary supplies for school, which are remarkably different to 'normal' school items.

Routledge
Taylor & Francis Group

WORKSHOP BREAKDOWNS

These workshop breakdowns are designed to show how to pick and choose ideas from the scripts in Part One and from the Explanation of Activities chapter, to create a drama from established themes and stories.

Using the 'Macbeth' workshop as an example, Act I: 'The Witches' Prophesies', is a reworking of 'Training Day'. Act II: 'Killing Duncan' is an adaptation of the game 'Grandmother's Footsteps' (p120). Act III: 'Banquo's Ghost' is a combination of the 'Run Away Boo!' activity (p123) and of 'Dragon Sleep', while Act IV: 'Further Riddles' and Act V: 'The Riddles Answered' repeat the format of the previous two acts, this time against Macbeth, rather than for him. The workshop breakdowns may also be used in conjunction with the scripts, for example, 'Under the Sea' could be a wonderful introduction to Shakespeare's 'The Tempest'.

Included at the end of Part Two are two 'Jack and the Beanstalk' workshop breakdowns. One is for use with more able participants and the other is a sensory workshop for those with profound and multiple learning difficulties (PMLD). Both are intended as a comprehensive introduction to leading a drama workshop, but again, they are simply a guide and should not be considered as the only way to lead a drama session.

MACBETH

These workshops are designed to introduce a group to Macbeth, by William Shakespeare, using text from the original script.

In this adaptation I have concentrated on the main plot developments for each act, which means they do vary in length (Act I is quite weighty compared with the rest). The intention was to explore moments from the script in chronological order, but not necessarily covering an entire act in one session.

NOTE: As this play involves witches, I have included them here. Some organisations I have worked with, however, take exception to witches and their association with the occult. If including the witches is too controversial, substitute their characters for that of a general narrator and focus the workshop more on the themes of ambition, greed and guilt. For example, cut the 'witchy' initiation or training in Act I, replace the hurly-burly dance with a sound orchestra of the battle or storm before meeting Macbeth and giving him the prophecy props. (See Act I, Scene ii in the original play for the text of the battle.)

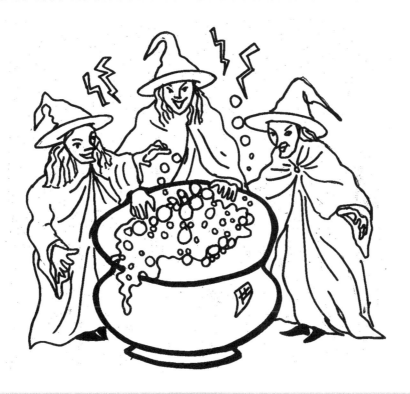

Character List

First Witch

Macbeth

Banquo (optional)

Duncan, King of Scotland
and his attendants

Ghost

Macduff

Props List

- Incense or an oil burner
- Cymbals, drums and other musical instruments
- Water mist spray
- Hurly-burly dance music (my suggestion, 'Summer' from *The Four Seasons* by Vivaldi)
- Witches' hat, hag costume or a collection of Halloween masks
- A broomstick (optional)
- Three prophecy picture props with appropriate text (see the craft note in the 'Additional Games and Activities' section for picture and text suggestions)
- Two medals
- A crown
- A large pot or cauldron (optional)
- Special ingredients (optional), such as rubber snakes, lizards and toads
- Three apparition picture props (see the craft note in the 'Additional Games and Activities' section for picture and text suggestions)
- A tree branch

WORKSHOP SCRIPT

Light incense or an oil burner before the group enters the room, to create a different smell there.

> **NOTE:** If necessary, do a character introduction such as the breakdown in the 'Dragon Sleep' script before taking on the role of First Witch.

Act I: The Witches' Prophecies

FIRST WITCH: When shall we three meet again

In thunder, lightning, or in rain?

Act I, Scene i

Use this rhyming couplet to interact with each participant. Repeat and use their names. Slow the speech down and use cymbals to punctuate the word thunder *and the water mist spray to create a sensation of rain.*

FIRST WITCH: As you all know, being a witch involves learning how to do various things.

Feel free to take suggestions from the group and extend or change their ideas accordingly.

FIRST WITCH: We have to learn how to …

- fly on our broomsticks

Demonstrate either with mime and/or a real broomstick.

- cast a spell

Make up some magic words and play the game 'Don't Move Until I Say'. Alternatively, use the spell to turn the group into various animals. See 'Animal Snap Cards' in the Explanation of Activities chapter.

- become invisible

Play an adaptation of the 'Compass Game'. If 'invisible' is shouted, the group must move as quickly as possible to that particular space. See the Explanation of Activities chapter for a description.

- cackle and laugh.

Routledge
Taylor & Francis Group

To complete their 'witchy' training, the participants dress up in costume, cackle and laugh. If there is only one witches' hat, costume or mask, share it by getting the participants to pass it on to the next person once they have completed their cackle.

FIRST WITCH: [name] When the hurly-burly's done,

When the battle's lost and won.

There to meet with Macbeth.

Encourage the group to laugh and cackle.

FIRST WITCH: Now the training is complete, let us enjoy ourselves.

Put on the hurly-burly music and dance about the room playing musical statues. Alternatively, create your own hurly-burly with a 'Sound Orchestra' (see the Explanation of Activities chapter) or create a storm such as in the 'Under the Sea' workshop breakdown. (The aim is to create a different pace or sensation between the hurly-burly dance and Macbeth's entrance.) During the paused moments in the hurly-burly dance, repeat the following dialogue.

FIRST WITCH: The heath is where we meet Macbeth.

And Banquo will be there.

We're going to tell them both three things.

So listen and beware.

Continue the hurlyburly dance for as long as necessary before Macbeth and Banquo enter.

FIRST WITCH: By the pricking of my thumbs,

Something wicked this way comes.

Act IV, Scene i

ALL WITCHES: Macbeth, Macbeth, Macbeth.

NOTE: If there is no one to play Macbeth, or you are demonstrating roles for the group to adopt, return the participants to their original places, drop the role of First Witch and describe the prophecies, (what each one is and what is going to happen). Give each prophecy prop to a person in the group; explain that you will now take on the role of Macbeth and that when you enter you will ask them if they have any news for him. That is their cue to then give you the picture props. Practise if necessary before taking on the actual role. If possible, choose someone to come with you as Banquo or cut the role and adapt his lines for Macbeth.

Routledge
Taylor & Francis Group

Macbeth and Banquo enter. Macbeth is wearing a medal.

MACBETH: So foul and fair a day I have not seen.

Banquo looks at the group of witches.

BANQUO: What are these?
So wither'd and so wild in their attire!

MACBETH: Speak, if you can: what are you?
Do you have anything for us?

Encourage the group to give you the prophecy picture props. It doesn't matter which order they are given in, but Macbeth reads the text and deciphers each.

MACBETH: What is this? A prophecy. For me?
All hail, Macbeth! Hail to thee, Thane of Glamis!
All hail, Macbeth! Hail to thee, Thane of Cawdor!
I hold the title Thane of Glamis already ...

He shows the group the medal he is wearing around his neck.

MACBETH: ... but I did not know I was going to be Thane of Cawdor! Do you have
anything else for me?

Encourage the group to give you another prophecy, which Macbeth reads.

MACBETH: All hail, Macbeth, thou shalt be king hereafter!
King! I would scarce believe it, but
If chance will have me king, why, chance may crown me,
Without my stir.

Act IV, Scene ii

NOTE: If guiding the group and teaching participants their dialogue, either get them to repeat dialogue directly after you or prompt with questions such as, 'Do you see these hags here? They look so wild. I wonder what they are?' This process of leading with questions and/or repeating dialogue in the scene can be applied to every character and even done during a presentation. Eventually, more able groups should be able to run the scene without your interference, however, if you are still concerned, make up dialogue cue cards with key words or phrases for the group to read.

This page may be photocopied for instructional use only. Drama Scripts for People with Special Needs © Sheree Vickers 2005

Routledge
Taylor & Francis Group

Macbeth asks the witches.

MACBETH: We already have a king of Scotland. King Duncan. How can I become king of Scotland if we have one already?

Repeat these questions to the group before encouraging them to give you another prophecy.

MACBETH: This is for you Banquo. It's a picture of your son, Fleance.

Banquo reads.

BANQUO: All hail, Banquo!

Lesser than Macbeth, and greater.

Not so happy, yet much happier.

Thou shalt get kings, though thou be none.

What does this mean ...

The witches cackle, laugh and exit (or return to their original places to watch the action).

BANQUO: ... whither are they vanish'd?

To Macbeth.

BANQUO: What does this mean?

MACBETH: Isn't it obvious? Your children shall be kings.

BANQUO: You shall be king.

MACBETH: And Thane of Cawdor too: went it not so?

BANQUO: Beware,

... oftentimes, to win us to our harm,

The instruments of darkness tell us truths.

Drop role and address the group as yourself, encouraging answers and reiterating the story so far.

NOTE: If using the script for a presentation, address these questions to the audience.

Routledge
Taylor & Francis Group

YOU: Do you think the witches are tricking Macbeth and Banquo? Do you think Macbeth will get another medal and become Thane of Cawdor? I wonder how he will become the king, because King Duncan is still alive. Here comes King Duncan now …

Cast Macbeth from the group and demonstrate the medal ceremony as King Duncan before repeating with different participants. Create a whole ceremony with Macbeth kneeling, the group clapping, trumpet calls and attendants creating an archway with their arms for King Duncan and Macbeth to walk under.

Duncan, King of Scotland, enters. He is wearing a crown.

DUNCAN: Worthy Macbeth! For an earnest of a greater honour,
I call thee Thane of Cawdor:

He places the second medal around Macbeth's neck.

DUNCAN: A banquet! Macbeth, we humbly beg your hospitality. Let us to your castle to feast and celebrate.

MACBETH: Sir, it would be my honour.

King Duncan and his attendants leave. Ask the participants to return to their original places and either reassume the role of Macbeth, or compare the prophecy picture prop of two medals with the ones around the neck of the participant playing Macbeth. Guide and adapt the dialogue as necessary.

MACBETH: Look, the prophecy has come true. I am Glamis and Thane of Cawdor. Look [name], the prophecy has come true …

He repeats (using the participants' names) and shows the medals to the group.

MACBETH: … and King Duncan comes to my castle tonight.
Well, if chance will have me king, why, chance may crown me,
Without my stir.

To the group or audience.

MACBETH: We already have a king. King Duncan. How can I become king if we have one already?

Repeat these questions to the group (allowing for various answers) before Macbeth exits.

Routledge
Taylor & Francis Group

Act II: Killing Duncan

It is night. If possible, change the lighting, music or smell in the room to denote a change of scene. Macbeth enters.

MACBETH: I have decided that the only way I am to become the king of Scotland is if I kill Duncan while he sleeps.

> **NOTE:** If the group is too scared, or is violently opposed to killing Duncan, change Macbeth's intention. Instead of killing Duncan, he is only going to steal his crown while he sleeps.

Set yourself up in a chair as the sleeping Duncan and adapt 'Grandmother's Footsteps'. Instead of having Duncan chase the group back, the participants must sneak up, steal his crown and run back themselves. If they succeed, reverse the roles and cast a participant as Duncan, with you sneaking up and speaking lines from the 'Is this a dagger...' speech. Continue to repeat and play before resuming the role of Macbeth.

MACBETH: Is this a dagger which I see before me,

The handle toward my hand? Come, let me clutch thee.

I have thee not, and yet I see thee still.

Act II, Scene i

Once Macbeth has the crown, compare it with the prophecy picture prop and address the group.

MACBETH: Look, the prophecy has come true. I am King of Scotland.

Repeat (using the participants' names) and show the crown to the group, possibly even allowing them to wear it, before taking it back, acting possessively and saying 'It's mine. I am the king'.

MACBETH: The prophecy has come true ... but what about Banquo? The witches said his son Fleance will be king.

Macbeth takes out the picture of Fleance wearing the crown and shows it to the group.

MACBETH: What am I to do about Banquo? Banquo's son is going to try and take my crown. What should I do?

He repeats these questions to the group (allowing for various answers) before he exits.

Act III: Banquo's Ghost

Return the room to its original state and address the group as yourself, reiterating the drama so far.

You: So, Macbeth is now king. He was wearing the crown. [Name], did you see him wearing the crown? Did he let you wear it? Everything the witches said has come true, but have you heard about the ghost? There is a ghost living in the castle and nobody knows who it is. He just appears. Who thinks they're brave enough to go and find out about the ghost?

Set up the space to play 'Run Away Boo!' (see the Explanation of Activities chapter).

You: This ghost is obviously scary, but I still wonder who it is. Who thinks they'd like to ask the ghost his name?

Guide the volunteer as you take on the role of the ghost yourself, with instructions such as, 'Remember, you can't run away this time. You have to ask the ghost his name'. When asked, the ghost replies.

GHOST: Banquo. My name is Banquo.

Drop role and remind the group who Banquo is.

You: Banquo. Do you remember him? He was Macbeth's friend. The witches said his son Fleance would be king.

Take out the picture prop and show them.

You: I wonder what happened to him. Shall we find out?

Choose a volunteer, remind him that he needs to ask what happened to Banquo and resume the role of Banquo's Ghost. Repeat or adapt the following dialogue as necessary.

GHOST: You want to know what happened to me? I was murdered. I was out riding my horse when three men attacked me. They were after my son Fleance, but he managed to escape. Do you want to know who murdered me? Macbeth.

The ghost exits. Address the group as yourself, reiterating the information.

You: Did you find out what happened to the ghost? Who killed him? Was it Macbeth? I wonder what Macbeth is up to now. Shall we find out? I think he's gone back to see the witches.

Act IV: Further Riddles

Set up the space for the witches as before. Have a large pot in the centre of the group (optional).

FIRST WITCH: Double, double toil and trouble;

Fire burn, and cauldron bubble.

Act IV, Scene i

Use this rhyming couplet to greet the group and review the witchy training again, reminding them to cackle and laugh. If the pot is available, have each participant add an ingredient to the pot.

FIRST WITCH: By the pricking of my thumbs,

Something wicked this way comes.

ALL WITCHES: Macbeth, Macbeth, Macbeth.

> **NOTE:** Encourage the witches to say 'Macbeth' at any time during this scene, either with electronic communication devices or incorporating a chant with stamping. See also 'Sound Orchestra' in the 'Explanation of Activities' chapter.

As before, drop the role of First Witch and describe these new apparitions. Show the group their double sides and explain that Macbeth can only see the 'Riddle' side. (Should the group refer to the other side, Macbeth can turn it over to look, but sees nothing.) Give each apparition prop to a person in the group, explain that you will now take on the role of Macbeth and when you enter you will ask them if they have any more news for him. That is their cue to then give you the picture props.

MACBETH: – I am in blood

Stepped in so far that, should I wade no more,

Returning were as tedious as go o'er:

Act III, Scene iv

I killed Duncan to get his crown and become king. I killed Banquo to stop his son Fleance from becoming king and even now I do not feel my crown is safe.

How now, you secret, black, and midnight hags!

– answer me

To what I ask you.

Act V, Scene i

Encourage the group to give you the apparition picture props. Macbeth reads the first apparition.

MACBETH: 'Macbeth! Macbeth! Macbeth! beware Macduff;

Beware the Thane of Fife.'

To the group.

MACBETH: Beware Macduff, but he is in England. What harm can he do me there?

Macbeth reads the second apparition.

MACBETH: 'Macbeth! Macbeth! Macbeth!

Be bloody, bold, and resolute; laugh to scorn

The power of man, for none of woman born

Shall harm Macbeth.'

To the group.

MACBETH: None of woman born! Everyone has a mother. This must mean that no one can harm me.

Macbeth reads the third apparition.

MACBETH: 'Macbeth shall never vanquish'd be until

Great Birnam wood to high Dunsinane hill

Shall come against him.'

To the group.

MACBETH: How can a wood full of trees march forward? Impossible.

Farewell, you secret, black, and midnight hags!

Macbeth exits. Encourage the group to cackle as you return the room to normal and readdress the participants as yourself.

YOU: So Macbeth needs to be careful of someone called Macduff. Do you know who Macduff is? He knows Macbeth took the crown away from Duncan and he knows that Macbeth killed Banquo. He's going to try and give the crown back to its rightful owner.

> **NOTE:** The aim of this discussion is to gain support for Macduff and to show how Macbeth 'play'dst most foully for' his crown and power.

YOU: So who would like to be Macduff?

Act V: The Riddles Answered

Cast Macduff, give him the tree branch to hide behind and instruct him to sneak up on Macbeth. (This is a repeat of 'Grandmother's Footsteps' and stealing Duncan's crown in Act II.) Mark a certain point on the floor for Macduff to stand on while Macbeth confronts him, and practise running back when Macbeth says 'Be gone!' If Macbeth falls down, they may take the crown.

Macbeth enters. Encourage the first Macduff to sneak up on him as practised.

MACBETH: What is this? I see a tree branch. Where is it from?

He looks at the apparition prop and reads the 'answer' side.

MACBETH: 'Macduff's army will cut down the trees in Birnam wood and march towards Macbeth's castle, holding the branches in front of them.' Is this tree from Birnam wood? I do not fear thee ... Be gone!

Chase Macduff back to his place. Drop role, recast Macduff and repeat the sneak-up.

MACBETH: Who are you? I see someone behind the tree branch.

He looks at the apparition prop and reads the riddle.

MACBETH: 'Macbeth! beware Macduff; Beware the Thane of Fife.'

Addressing the sneaking participant.

MACBETH: Are you Macduff? Are you trying to get my crown back?
Well you can't have it.
I bear a charmed life, which must not yield,
To one of woman born.

Act V, Scene viii

I do not fear thee. Be gone!

Chase Macduff back to his place. Drop role, recast Macduff and repeat the sneak-up. Remind the group that if Macbeth falls down they may get his crown. (Remind the participants also to be careful where they step, ie, not to step on Macbeth's head!)

MACBETH: The witches said beware Macduff and here Macduff comes. The witches said that Birnam wood would walk and here I see the wood. Yet none of woman born shall harm Macbeth.

Routledge
Taylor & Francis Group

He looks at the third apparition prop, reading the 'answer' side.

MACBETH: What is this?

'Macduff was not born naturally. He was born caesarean. His mother needed help from a doctor.'

Out, out, brief candle!

Life's but a walking shadow, a poor player

That struts and frets his hour upon the stage

And then is heard no more: it is a tale

Told by an idiot, full of sound and fury,

Signifying nothing.

Act V, Scene v

Macbeth falls down and the group gets his crown back. Finish with a discussion on whether Macbeth should have taken it in the first place. Whose fault it was (his or the witches') and who the rightful owner should be now.

Further ideas for a sensory workshop

◎ Use a mirror to show the group their transformation into witches.

◎ Add scarves and streamers into the hurly-burly dance.

◎ Actually cook a meal in the pot for the witches' apparitions in Act IV.

◎ Use actual props, for example, medals, a crown and a doll for Banquo's son Fleance, rather than picture representations for the prophecies and apparitions.

Additional games and activities

◎ Include Macbeth's 'Is this a dagger …' speech (see Shakespeare's original text, Act II, Scene i) and play a 'Dagger Grab' game. Hang a picture representation of a dagger with fishing line from a piece of dowelling, and as the text is spoken, the group tries to grab it. (Have them sitting down to play this game, if it becomes too boisterous.)

◎ Make up your own witch spell or recipe. What ingredients would they put in their spell? Compare it with the original text in Act IV, Scene i.

◎ In this workshop script the character of Lady Macbeth has been deliberately cut (to focus more on Macbeth's relationship to the prophecies and the witches' interference), therefore spend a session looking at Macbeth's relationship with his wife and how his behaviour and choices also lead to her downfall. (See Act V, Scene i, in the original play for text relating to Lady Macbeth's decline.)

◎ Have they ever wanted something belonging to somebody else?

Three prophecy picture props

◎ A picture of two medals with the following text:

> All hail, Macbeth! Hail to thee, Thane of Glamis!
> All hail, Macbeth! Hail to thee, Thane of Cawdor!

◎ A picture of a crown with the following text:

> All hail, Macbeth, thou shalt be king hereafter!

A picture of a child wearing a crown with the following text:

> *All hail, Banquo!*
>
> *Lesser than Macbeth, and greater.*
>
> *Not so happy, yet much happier.*
>
> *Thou shalt get kings, though thou be none.*

Three apparition picture props

These picture props need to be double-sided. One side is marked 'Riddle', the other side 'Answer'. Cover the 'Answer' side in glitter to give it a different texture.

First Apparition

On the 'Riddle' side is a picture of a sword with the following text:

> *'Macbeth! Macbeth! Macbeth! Beware Macduff;*
>
> *Beware the Thane of Fife.'*

On the 'Answer' side the following text:

> *Macduff has fled to England and is preparing an army to invade Scotland and take the crown away from Macbeth.*

Second Apparition

On the 'Riddle' side is a picture of a woman with the following text:

> *'Macbeth! Macbeth! Macbeth!*
>
> *Be bloody, bold, and resolute; laugh to scorn*
>
> *The power of man, for none of woman born*
>
> *Shall harm Macbeth.'*

On the 'Answer' side the following text:

> *Macduff was not born naturally. He was born caesarean. His mother needed help from a doctor.*

NOTE: Details of a caesarean birth can be expanded or explained at your discretion.

This page may be photocopied for instructional use only. Drama Scripts for People with Special Needs • Sheree Vickers 2005

Third Apparition

On the 'Riddle' side is a picture of a woman with the following text:

> *'Macbeth shall never vanquish'd be until*
> *Great Birnam wood to high Dunsinane hill*
> *Shall come against him.'*

On the 'Answer' side the following text:

> *Macduff's army will cut down the trees in Birnam wood and march*
> *towards Macbeth's castle, holding the branches in front of them.*

GOBONZO'S HYPNOTIST SHOW

This workshop has been used with a variety of ages and abilities, and it is guaranteed to provide a fun session exploring different music and dance styles.

Character List

The Great Gobonzo

Trixi his assistant

Participants in the audience

Props List

- Cape for Gobonzo

- A wig or feather boa for Trixi

- A fob watch, whistle or some form of swinging pendulum prop

- A fanfare for Gobonzo's entrance

- Special audiotape made up with different genres of music, from Elvis Presley to medieval minstrel music

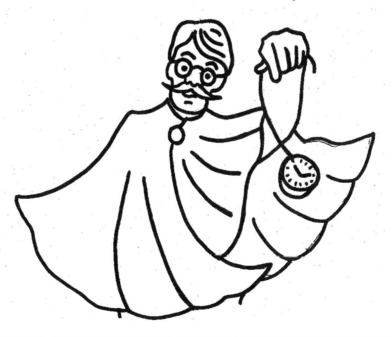

WORKSHOP SCRIPT

Entrance fanfare music for Gobonzo that ends abruptly.

GOBONZO: Good evening ladies and gentlemen. I am 'The Great Gobonzo'.

Gobonzo bows with a flourish. Hopefully the group will clap. If not, encourage them to do so.

GOBONZO: That's right. When I bow, you all need to clap your hands like this ...

He demonstrates.

GOBONZO: Let me try again.

Re-enter to the fanfare music and bow with a flourish.

GOBONZO: Thank you.

Drop role and address the group.

YOU: Would anyone else like to be Gobonzo?

Dress a volunteer in Gobonzo's cape and direct him to enter and bow to mountainous applause.

YOU: Here's your cape. Come over here and, when the music starts, walk to here ...

Possibly mark a cross on the floor with chalk or tape.

YOU: ... and do a big bow like this ...

Demonstrate.

YOU: ... so everyone can clap. Ready? Wait for the music ... go!

Put the fanfare music back on and guide participants through the above process. When all the Gobonzos have finished, take the role back on yourself.

GOBONZO: Wonderful! We've all bowed to the fanfare music, and so now it's time to introduce my assistant Trixi.

Calling for her.

GOBONZO: Trixi? Trixi, where are you? She's got my watch. I can't hypnotise without my watch. Let me go and find her.

Exit as Gobonzo and re-enter as Trixi (or cast a participant as Trixi).

TRIXI: Sorry I'm late. I'm Trixi!

She curtseys.

TRIXI: Have you met Gobonzo yet? He's going to try and hypnotise you all. He has this watch ...

She produces the fob watch.

TRIXI: ... that he waves like this ...

Trixi swings the fob watch back and forth.

TRIXI: ... and says 'You are all getting sleepy. You will do everything I say'. And then he claps his hands and tells us all to do things. Shall we practise?

Swinging the fob watch.

TRIXI: You are all getting sleepy, now everybody ...

Clap your hands.

TRIXI: ... sit up straight.

Encourage the group to sit up very straight.

TRIXI: Everybody ...

Clap your hands.

TRIXI: ... pull a funny face.

Make up a list and take suggestions from the group as to other hypnotic activities. Ask various participants to clap their hands and lead the group. When everyone has finished practising, Trixi readdresses the group.

TRIXI: I'd better go and tell Gobonzo I'm here now. Who would like to look after the swinging watch?

Give the watch to a participant.

TRIXI: Ensure that you give that to Gobonzo when he comes back in. Bye everyone. Have fun.

Trixi exits as Gobonzo re-enters.

NOTE: If able to cast both roles, develop the following scene for both of them to lead.

GOBONZO: Where is my watch? Has Trixi given you my watch yet?

Encourage the group to give you back the watch.

GOBONZO: Did she show you how to use it? Wonderful, then we can start!

Ladies and gentlemen, I am 'The Great Gobonzo' and I am here to hypnotise you all.

He claps his hands and repeats the list of hypnotic activities with the group.

GOBONZO: And now … I have here a very special tape. We need to listen closely. As each different piece of music is played, each of you will dance in a different way.

Play the tape of music and take dance or movement suggestions for each different style, for example start swinging hips like Elvis Presley, clucking like chickens for 'Old MacDonald', etc. Have the participants dance individually, in pairs or as a whole group.

> **NOTE:** Take your time over developing the movement or dance activities. Stop the tape at any time to try different suggestions and build the act up slowly with the group.

End the tape with a lullaby that sends the group to sleep.

Routledge
Taylor & Francis Group

Further ideas for a sensory workshop

- Adapt the hypnotic activities depending on the abilities of the group, for example, spin around, blow bubbles and smile. The swinging pendulum could be a mobile of sensory props that is accompanied by the following poem:

  > *Count to three and clap your hands*
  > *One, two, three!*
  > *The Great Gobonzo makes demands*
  > *I wonder what they'll be?*

- Hypnotise each participant with glitter. Use their names, count to three and blow glitter over each.

- Explore each piece of music with a related prop, for example 'Old MacDonald Had a Farm' could involve feathers, fur and drinking milk; Chinese music could involve dancing with silk scarves or the playing of instruments with chopsticks.

Additional games and activities

- Try looking at some other simple magic tricks or optical illusions.

- Develop the hypnotist act into a full variety event, with participants showing off skills in other areas, such as singing their favourite song, playing an instrument or performing a short skit.

Routledge
Taylor & Francis Group

BABOUSHKA

In a multicultural and multi-faith society, this traditional Russian folk-tale can be explored without the Christmas story if necessary.

Character List

Narrator

Baboushka

The kings

NOTE: Although traditionally the story has three kings, the number can vary from one to the whole group.

Props List

- A torch

- Cardboard with the shape of a cut-out star (put over the torchlight and shone on the ceiling it creates a shining star)

- Apron or shawl for Baboushka

- A crown for the king

- A copy of Brahms' Lullaby

- A note with the following written on it: 'Baboushka, thank you for your hospitality. We are following the star in search of a new king. Would you like to come with us?'

- A basket full of treats, such as Christmas crackers, stickers or miniature chocolates

- Pen and paper (to create a list of wishes and clean-up activities)

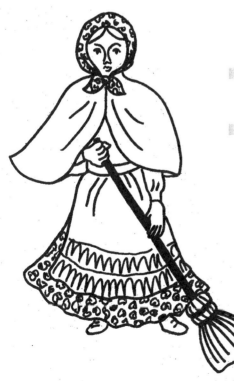

WORKSHOP SCRIPT

Scene I: Star Light, Star Bright

Sing the song 'Twinkle, Twinkle Little Star'.

> *Twinkle, twinkle little star*
> *How I wonder where you are.*
> *Up above the world so high*
> *Like a diamond in the sky.*
> *Twinkle, twinkle little star*
> *How I wonder where you are.*

NARRATOR:　　There was an amazing star in the sky. It was brighter than all the other stars. Can you see it?

Darken the room and use the torch and cardboard cut-out to shine the star shape around the room.

> **NOTE:** If you are unable to use a dark room, try using a mirror to reflect sunshine or have someone hold up a handmade, sparkly, cut-out star.

NARRATOR:　　All the villagers came out to see the amazing star.

> *Star light, star bright*
> *First star I see tonight.*
> *Wish I may, wish I might*
> *Have the wish I wish tonight?*

Repeat the rhyme asking participants what they would wish for.

NARRATOR:　　If you could wish upon a star, what would you wish?

Make a list of all the wishes.

Routledge
Taylor & Francis Group

NARRATOR: Do you know who would like to see the star? Baboushka. We should tell Baboushka about the star. Do you know who Baboushka is? She's very busy. She has to clean her house and make toys for the village children. Let's go and see what she's up to.

Scene II: Cleaning the House

Put Baboushka's shawl on and introduce her character. (See the 'Dragon Sleep' script for a breakdown on introducing a new character to a nervous group.)

BABOUSHKA: Hello everyone. It's lovely of you to come visit me. Why are you here?

> **NOTE:** Prompt with questions such as, 'Is there something in the sky? I've heard about an amazing star that's been shining more brightly than the others. Have you all been making wishes?', etc.

BABOUSHKA: I'd love to come and look at the star but I have to finish my cleaning. Would you like to help me?

> **NOTE:** Should the group say 'No', continue to clean the house yourself, getting suggestions for activities from them.

Play the 'Clean-Up Mime' activity (see the Explanation of Activities chapter). During the activity, choose someone else to be Baboushka, put the shawl on him and lead the group with 'We have a new Baboushka. Baboushka, what shall we clean?' The new Baboushka then chooses another clean-up activity from the list (or makes one up himself). Repeat with multiple Baboushkas and activities until the house is clean.

BABOUSHKA: Thank you all so much for helping me clean my house, but I'm afraid I still can't come and see the amazing star. I have loads of toys to make.

Return everyone to their place ready to make some toys.

Scene III: Toy making

BABOUSHKA: I make all the toys for the village children. Would you like to help me? What toy would you like to make? What's your favourite toy?

Ask individual participants to show you the actions for their toy. Ask the rest of the group to copy the action.

This page may be photocopied for instructional use only. *Drama Scripts for People with Special Needs* © Sheree Vickers 2005

Routledge
Taylor & Francis Group

NOTE: Try and make a distinction between playing *with* the toy and *being* the toy. For example, if the participants are playing with a bouncing ball, jump around the room as the actual ball. If they are playing with a train, make a long 'follow-the-leader' line and create train noises. Alternatively, if flying a kite, it might be easier to do the action of holding on to the string.

BABOUSHKA: Thank you all so much for helping me make all the toys for the village children. Now I can come and see the amazing star in the sky.

Darken the room, sing 'Twinkle, Twinkle Little Star' and repeat the star effect with the torch and cardboard cut-out for Baboushka.

BABOUSHKA: How beautiful. I'm so glad you showed me the star. It really was amazing, but it's very late now, so I'd better go to bed. Goodnight.

Give Baboushka's shawl to a participant and have him go to sleep in a corner of the room before returning to the role of Narrator.

Scene IV: The Kings' Visit

NARRATOR: Baboushka was fast asleep when there was a knocking at the door.

NOTE: This next sequence is an adaptation of 'Snore Sshh!' (see the Explanation of Activities chapter) and can be set up in a practice session, guiding the sleeping Baboushka into saying 'Sshh!' after each set of knocking.

The kings enter, speak loudly and mime the action of knocking on a door.

KINGS: Knock, knock, knock.

BABOUSHKA: Sshh!

KINGS: Knock, knock, knock.

BABOUSHKA: Sshh!

Repeat with many Baboushkas and play around with the dialogue, for example change the 'Knock, knock, knock!' to 'We want to come in' or 'Anybody home?' etc.

NARRATOR: Finally, Baboushka answered the door and what do you think she saw?

Give the king's crown to a participant and have the group bow as they enter the space. (Alternatively let the whole group wear their pre-made crowns.) Sing the carol 'We Three Kings'. During the carol, take back Baboushka's shawl and resume the role.

> *We three kings of Orient are*
> *Bearing gifts we traverse afar*
> *Field and fountain, moor and mountain*
> *Following yonder star.*
>
> *O star of wonder, star of night*
> *Star with royal beauty bright*
> *Westward leading, still proceeding*
> *Guide us to thy perfect light.*

BABOUSHKA: Your majesties. Are you following that amazing star in the sky? I saw it too. It was beautiful. Please come in and rest your heads.

Welcome the group into your house. Use their names and bow to each participant.

BABOUSHKA: I'm afraid I don't have much food in the house, but what I do have I'll happily share with you.

Use the following rhyme to encourage each member of the group to tell you what their favourite food is. Expand by adapting the memory game 'I Went To The Shop' (see the Explanation of Activities chapter).

> *Will you share some food with me, food with me, food with me?*
> *Will you share some food with me? Let's eat now!*
>
> *My favourite food is [ice cream], [ice cream], [ice cream]*
> *My favourite food is [ice cream]. What is yours?*
>
> *Her/His favourite food is [new food], etc.*

Once this activity is finished, yawn loudly.

BABOUSHKA: My goodness. It's very late. I think it's time for bed. Goodnight everyone.

Remove Baboushka's shawl and play Brahms' Lullaby or say a nursery rhyme as you move the group back to their original places. Ask the participants to remove their crowns and choose someone to leave a note behind on the ground.

NARRATOR: In the morning the kings were gone, but they had left Baboushka a note.

Routledge
Taylor & Francis Group

Resume Baboushka's role or guide someone else in the role as she reads the note.

BABOUSHKA: 'Baboushka, thank you for your hospitality. We are following the star in search of a new king. Would you like to come with us?'

To the group.

BABOUSHKA: I would love to go with them, but I'm so busy. I have the beds to make and the floors to sweep and more toys to make. Maybe if I work really hard I can meet the kings later.

Repeat the 'Clean-Up Mime' activities, asking the group for help in remembering what was on the list.

BABOUSHKA: Now that I've finished the cleaning, I can get my basket and fill it full of treats for the new king.

Remove Baboushka's shawl and address the group as the Narrator.

NARRATOR: Baboushka packed up her basket full of treats and went in search of the kings. She went to village after village, asking about them, but she never found them. However, every time she saw a smiling, happy child she gave them one of the treats from her basket.

Repeat sections of the above dialogue as necessary before picking up the basket of treats and resuming the role of Baboushka.

BABOUSHKA: Hello [name], I'm looking for the kings that came to visit. Have you seen them?

> **NOTE:** It doesn't matter what the answer is to this question. If the group answers 'No', act disappointed, if the answer is 'Yes', ask for directions before continuing with the scene.

BABOUSHKA: Would you like a treat from my basket? Can you smile for me?

Encourage them to smile and laugh.

BABOUSHKA: Wonderful.

Give each participant a treat and end with the Christmas carol 'We Wish You A Merry Christmas'.

> We wish you a merry Christmas
> We wish you a merry Christmas
> We wish you a merry Christmas
> And a happy New Year
>
> Good tidings we bring
> To you and your kin
> We wish you a merry Christmas
> And a happy New Year.

Routledge
Taylor & Francis Group

Further ideas for a sensory workshop

- In a safe environment, use sparklers or candles for each starlight wish, or use a special sound, such as the tinkles from a xylophone.

- Actually wish for some things that could appear, for example a chocolate cake or a special toy.

- Using a feather duster, damp face-cloth and small washing-up mop, play the 'Clean-Up Mime' with each participant by actually cleaning them or the area immediately surrounding them. Alternatively, play the 'Wash Rinse Spin Stop' game (see the Explanation of Activities chapter).

- Have a box of different toys for the group to play with, such as a bouncing ball, a doll, a racing car, a train, etc. Explore each with the following rhyme.

  I'm making all the toys
  For all the girls and boys.
  Some are soft and some are round
  And each makes such a different sound.
  (Oh look, here we have a [name of toy]
  I wonder what sound it makes?)

- Use the following traditional rhyme for the king's entrance.

  Knock at the door.

  Tap the participant's forehead or back of the hand.

  Ring the bell.

  Gently tug at the participant's earlobe.

  Lift the latch.

  Gently pinch the participant's nose.

  And walk in.

  Tickle the lips with your fingers or pitter-pat your fingers up his arm.

- Have a little Christmas feast prepared for the kings' visit, even popping Christmas crackers.

Additional games and activities

◎ Dress up as the villagers from Baboushka's home and create a marketplace scene. (See the 'Jack and the Beanstalk' workshop breakdown for ideas on how to do this.) Decorate the village square with decorations.

◎ Create a starry mobile. Write down everybody's wish on his or her individual star.

◎ Spend a session making crowns.

◎ Use a Russian doll to set the scene and location of the folk-tale. Compare this doll with modern or western-style dolls. Explore the history of the story by referring to how she would have cleaned the house, for example not having a vacuum cleaner or washing machine.

Routledge
Taylor & Francis Group

UNDER THE SEA

This tactile adventure was first worked with participants who had profound and multiple learning difficulties (PMLD). There were seven members of the group (aged between 9 and 14); all were in wheelchairs and in a very restricted space.

Character List

Seagull

Octopus

Mermaid

> **NOTE:** I originally used a seagull puppet as the group's guide, but it could be a more neutral role or any character related to the beach.

Props List

- Seagull puppet or feathers
- Sound-effect tape of water lapping (if unavailable, use music appropriate to the beach)
- Non-allergenic sunscreen or moisture cream (optional)
- Sun hats (optional)
- Containers of fine porridge oats for sand
- A collection of shells (buried in the sand containers)

more items overleaf

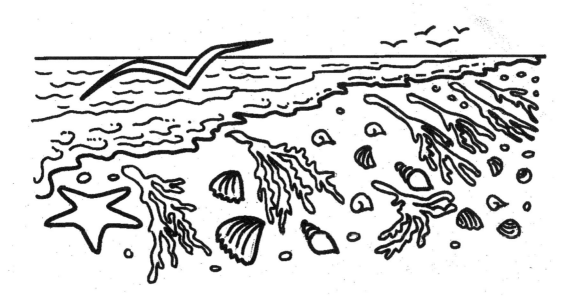

Props List *(continued)*

- Bucket and spade (optional)

- Wet wool for seaweed (wet with salty water)

- A beach ball

- A picture of a boat

- Newspaper sailor hats for each participant

- Balloons or a set of water wings

- A salt-water mist spray

- A piece of classical music to represent under the water (my suggestion, Fauré's *Pavane*)

- Lamp and blue scarf (optional)

- Bubble mix for blowing bubbles

- A collection of tinfoil fish and fishing-line (see craft note in 'Additional Games and Activities' section for details on how to make these)

- An octopus puppet prop (use clothes-pegs to attach long lengths of streamers to a wire coat-hanger or hula hoop, and add some large eyes at the top)

- A tambourine

- A crown for the mermaid (make from some shiny cardboard and glitter)

- A long roll of bubble-wrap

- Blue or black material for a 'Parachute Run'

WORKSHOP SCRIPT

Seagull greets everyone in the group.

SEAGULL: Skwark! Hello [name], are you coming to the beach with me? I live at the beach. Skwark! I'm a seagull. I like to fly high in the air and out to sea. I'm flying out to sea to look for my friend the whale. He doesn't come round much anymore and I miss him. I'm going to look for him under the sea, but first we have to go to the beach. Have you ever been to the beach? There's sand and salty water and shells and seaweed. Would you like to come? Skwark! Hello [name], are you coming to the beach with me? [name] is coming. I'm a seagull ...

Repeat until the entire group has been welcomed.

> **NOTE:** The above opening paragraph is extremely 'wordy'. Depending on the group, streamline the text by picking out key phrases or replacing some words with feathery textures, music or sounds.

SEAGULL: Skwark! We are all going to the beach, but we can't go to the beach without putting on our sunscreen and wearing our sun hats.

Put on the water-lapping sounds tape. Wear sun hats and rub sunscreen onto each participant's hands and/or face (as appropriate) while saying the following rhyme.

> *Sunshine, sunshine*
> *All through the day*
> *Sunshine, sunshine*
> *As we go out to play.*
> *Sunshine, sunshine*
> *On our merry way*
> *Sunshine, sunshine*
> *Never go away.*

SEAGULL: Skwark! Welcome to the beach everyone. Shall we play on the sand? Who can find some shells?

Routledge
Taylor & Francis Group

Take out containers of porridge oats and look for the various shells. Pad the oats down and create patterns of different footprints (for example, crabs, birds and humans). Use the wet, woolly seaweed to brush across their hands and faces. As the participants are playing in the 'sand', show various discoveries to others in the group.

> **NOTE:** Fine porridge oats are a good option, as they cause no harm if eaten. However, their texture doesn't allow the creation of sandcastles. If sand is available, extend this section with a sandcastle building competition.

SEAGULL: Skwark! What have you found there [name]? A shell? May I take it over to [name] and show them? Skwark! Look at this shell. If you listen into it, you can hear the sea.

Hold a shell up to the participants' ears.

SEAGULL: Skwark! [name], can you hear the sea?

> **NOTE:** By referring to others in the group, it emphasises that the drama they are participating in is a collective experience. It also promotes sharing.

When finished playing in the sand and with the shells, pack them away and blow up the beach ball.

SEAGULL: Skwark! Look at this. A beach ball. Shall we play? Skwark! Don't let it touch the ground. Can we keep it in the air?

Bounce the large beach ball around the group.

SEAGULL: Skwark! Guess what everybody – I see a boat. We need to put on our sailor hats.

Show everyone the picture of a boat. Sing the 'Sailor Went To Sea Song' (see the Explanation of Activities chapter) while putting newspaper sailor hats on each participant.

SEAGULL: Now before anyone can go on to the water, we have to put on our life-jackets. Skwark!

If available, use a set of blow-up water wings on each participant, otherwise play 'Letting Go Fizzle' (see 'Balloon Tricks' in the Explanation of Activities chapter) to demonstrate.

SEAGULL: Everyone put your life-jackets on. If you need to use them you pull this little tab here and they blow up really big.

Demonstrate being inflated with the balloon.

SEAGULL: Uh oh, skwark! Help me someone.

Go up to a member of the group.

SEAGULL: Could you help me deflate my life-jacket? Just push that little button there.

The imaginary button, once pressed, fizzles the balloon around the room. If available, an electronic communication device can be used, not just for the life-jacket button, but for all sorts of under-sea sounds.

SEAGULL: Skwark! Skwark! Skwark! Oh no, let's try that again.

Repeat the 'Letting Go Fizzle' exercise with each participant.

SEAGULL: I think we're now ready to go out onto the water in our boat. Skwark! Be careful everyone. The salty water likes to splash as we row.

Say the following rhyme while spraying the participant's faces with the salt-water mist spray.

SEAGULL: Skwark! [name], can you taste the salty sea water?

> *Water spraying, water spraying*
> *Salt is in the air.*
> *Lick your lips and breathe it in,*
> *Taste it everywhere.*

SEAGULL: Now that we're in our boat on the sea, can anyone see my friend the whale? He's very big and he swims in the sea. Can anyone see him? Skwark! He doesn't come round much anymore and I miss him. I think we're going to have to go for a swim in the sea to find him. [name], would you like to go for a swim to look for my friend the whale?

Repeat as necessary.

SEAGULL: Get ready to dive into the water everyone. Hold your breath ... and ... dive!

Turn the lights off (if possible, create a blue light effect by putting a coloured scarf over a lamp) and change the music.

This page may be photocopied for instructional use only. Drama Scripts for People with Special Needs © Sheree Vickers 2005

> **NOTE:** Should any members of the group protest to the dive, saying they either won't be able to hold their breath for that long, or are worried about breathing, get Seagull to discover a magic spell that can make them all breath underwater.

SEAGULL: Skwark! I love going down under the sea. Can you see the bubbles?

Blow bubbles to individuals in the group. If possible, move the group in and around the bubbles to the music.

SEAGULL: The ocean is full of wonderful animals. Let's see if we can catch some fish.

Swim some tinfoil fish around before bringing out the magnet fishing-line and catching them.

SEAGULL: Do we all have some fish? Skwark! I love eating fish. While we were fishing, did anyone see my friend the whale? He's very big and he swims in the sea. Skwark! He doesn't come round much anymore and I miss him. [name], did you see him at all?

Repeat as necessary.

SEAGULL: We'll have to keep looking ... Uh oh, skwark! Look who's coming. It's Octopus. He likes to catch people in his tentacles.

Use the long streamer tentacles and tambourine to denote Octopus.

OCTOPUS: Well, well, well. Who do we have swimming here? I see you've all been fishing. I like to fish too. I wonder who I'll catch in my tentacles?

> *Swimming, swimming in the sea.*
> *Like the fishes do.*
> *Careful, careful as you swim*
> *Or I'll catch ... you!*

On 'You', drop Octopus's tentacles over someone. Repeat the rhyme and game with each participant.

OCTOPUS: Why, why, why are you all swimming in the sea? Mermaid will know. Let me go and get Mermaid.

Octopus exits.

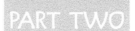
> **NOTE:** If playing all three roles of Seagull, Octopus and Mermaid, have one character leave before the other enters. Alternatively, have Seagull stay with the group, joining in with interactions and helping to guide the group in each activity.

SEAGULL: Skwark! Has anyone found my friend the whale yet? He's very big and he swims in the sea. Skwark! He doesn't come round much anymore and I miss him.

Continue to ask each participant.

SEAGULL: Skwark! Look who's coming. It's Mermaid. She's beautiful. She might know where Whale is.

Mermaid enters wearing her beautiful crown.

MERMAID: Welcome to my underwater kingdom. I see you've been fishing and have met Octopus, but you're still looking for the wonderful whale. There is only one way to meet Whale. We have to close our eyes and call him by going 'Sshh'!

Mermaid demonstrates.

MERMAID: Can we all do that?

Encourage the participants to close their eyes and make the 'Sshh!!' sound. Dim the lights further and turn the music off.

MERMAID: Here comes Whale. Sshh!

Unroll the bubble-wrap and, as the group continues to make the sound, brush the bubble-wrap across their arms, legs and faces.

MERMAID: Whale doesn't come round much anymore. All his family and friends were hunted for their blubber and now there are very few left. Sshh!

Once Whale has visited everybody, put the underwater music and lighting back on.

MERMAID: You can open your eyes now everyone. Whale has gone. I'm going to have to take you all back to the beach, but I'm afraid a storm is coming. We can only escape the storm by running under the waves when they are high in the air. Let me show you.

This page may be photocopied for instructional use only *Drama Scripts for People with Special Needs* © Sheree Vickers 2005

Routledge
Taylor & Francis Group

> **NOTE:** This poem and the accompanying 'Parachute Run' (see the Explanation of Activities chapter) are wonderful for creating tension. Feel free to add a long pause between the two stanzas.

Stanza one is spoken very calmly and quietly, with the material wafting gently.

> A storm is coming
>
> Hear it creep
>
> The sea is calm
>
> Don't make a peep.

Stanza two is spoken loudly and angrily, with the material vigorously waving in the air to create a wonderfully windy effect.

> The sea grows wild
>
> Waves cover the sun
>
> We need to take cover,
>
> Ready, steady ... RUN!

On 'Run', individuals escape under the waved material (either running through it themselves or having the material moved over them). When everyone is through the storm, return the lights to normal beach mode and put the water-lapping sounds tape back on.

SEAGULL: Skwark! I'm so glad you all managed to escape the storm. Thank you all for coming to the beach and helping me find my friend whale. Did you feel him swim by? He's very big. He's the biggest creature on the planet and he swims in the sea.

End by singing the 'Sailor Went To Sea Song' again, substituting 'a sailor' with the names of those in the group.

Routledge
Taylor & Francis Group

Further ideas for a sensory workshop

- Use a fan to create an outside breeze.

- Put on sunglasses to escape the sun's glare. A torch shone on the face can create the sensation of the sun.

- If you have access to a black room with fluorescent lights, this workshop makes full use of those ideal facilities during the underwater dive.

- Pull some fishy faces in a mirror.

- Eat some ice cream or have some fish and chips at the end of the adventure (relate back to the fish you caught under the sea).

Additional games and activities

- Create a sandy collage of shells, seaweed and footprints in containers to display, or use a piece of net curtain to make a textured display of fish, coral and other underwater inhabitants.

- Find some tin cans and other items of rubbish on the beach and explore the environmental cost of pollution. For example, oil-slicks and their effect on seals and birds, or the cost of certain fishing-nets on species such as dolphin.

- Go on a wildlife conservation trek to find other endangered species, such as a trip to China to find the panda, or Africa to find the elephant.

- Create a list of rules for sailing on the boat or swimming in the water.

- Discover a pirate ship on the ocean or induct everyone as mermaids, getting them to make their own crowns to wear.

Tinfoil fish

Cut out fish shapes from tinfoil. Hang them with some fishing-line from a piece of dowelling and 'swim' them around the room. Brush the tinfoil fish with tuna or sardine oil to give them a fishy smell. Different coloured card, cellophane or wrapping paper also work well. To go fishing, add paper-clips to each tinfoil fish, place them on the ground and create a fishing-line with a magnet on the end. The magnet should then attract the paper-clip fish.

Routledge
Taylor & Francis Group

JACK AND THE BEANSTALK

First worked over four, two-hour sessions with a group of autistic children, aged between 8 and 14 years.

Props List

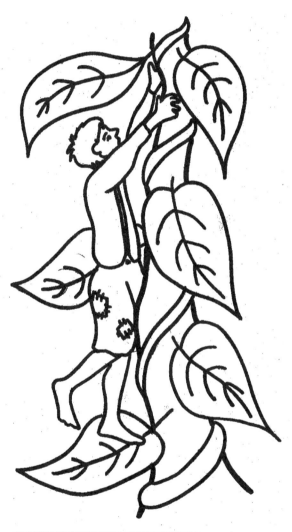

- Apron for the shopkeeper
- Beans (pumpkin seeds or picture representations)
- Golden eggs (hard-boiled and sprayed with gold paint)
- Shop props (for example, actual cans of food or picture card representations, real pennies, or paper money)
- Rope
- Bird puppet, a feather boa or a feather duster
- Servant's hat or other character prop
- Parachute material
- A drum

NOTE: Dad, older sister or brother can replace the character of Mum. Occasionally, the character has also been Foster Mum. As these roles can hold significance for the participants, it is fine to adapt them as necessary. Daisy the Cow has even turned into Daisy the Elephant, Hamster and Lizard.

Character List

Narrator	Servant
Jack	Goosey
Mum	Daisy the Cow
Customers in the shop	Shopkeeper

WORKSHOP SCRIPT

NARRATOR: This is the story of 'Jack and the Beanstalk'. Do you know the story of 'Jack and the Beanstalk'? Well, it goes like this ...

> **NOTE:** Asking a question such as 'Do you know the story of "Jack and the Beanstalk"?' can prompt some in the group into storytelling, where they may want to share their own 'Jack and the Beanstalk' tale. Allow them to continue with this (even though at times the story may be completely unrecognisable from the original) because it helps to empower the participants with the concept, is a lovely way to get to know the group and it also allows them to be in the 'spotlight'. If, however, you have limited time, steer the drama back with a simple phrase such as 'Can you remember it and tell me later?', or if they insist (and by not telling their story it will cause a distraction and make it impossible for them to fully participate in the drama), allow them to tell it or pass them over to a helper who can listen.

Scene I: Introducing Jack

NARRATOR: Jack didn't want to go to bed because he'd had no food.

JACK: I don't want to go to bed. I've had no food!

MUM: We need to go to market to get some food. But we've got no money. We'd better sell the Daisy the Cow.

DAISY: Moo!

JACK: Come on Daisy. Let's go to market.

DAISY: Moo!

> **NOTE:** Cast the drama during the storytelling, for example, 'Jack didn't want to go to bed ... who wants to be Jack?, or 'Would you like to say "I don't want to go to bed?"', etc. This is the perfect way to demonstrate and guide and can be simplified and repeated with as many Jacks and mums as necessary.

Everyone gets ready to go to market by singing songs, for example, 'The Wheels on the Bus', or by playing games such as 'Follow-the-Leader'. Eventually everyone arrives at the market.

Scene II: The Marketplace

NARRATOR: We're here now!

> **NOTE:** Before continuing with the drama, sit everyone down again and prepare them for the next scene. The marketplace can be established by setting up a table and putting on an apron. (See 'Setting Up The Space' and 'Taking On A Role' in the 'Introduction'.) Guide with questions such as 'Who's been shopping before?', 'What did you buy?', etc. For those that find imagination and 'pretend' items difficult to comprehend, use the collected shop props and pennies. Demonstrate both the role of the shopkeeper and the customer for the group.

SHOPKEEPER: Hello [name]. Welcome to my shop. In this shop you can buy anything you want.

Give some examples, such as food, clothes, a pet animal, etc, although guiding too much can lead the participants to copy your suggestions rather than using their own imaginations.

SHOPKEEPER: What would you like to buy?

CUSTOMER 1: [item]

SHOPKEEPER: Would you like a big [item] or a small [item]?

CUSTOMER 1: [response]

> **NOTE:** For visual clarity, big items should be stored on one side of the shop and small items on the other. Alternatively, move the participants' hands to demonstrate big and small, whilst saying the various items, for example big sausages, little sausages, etc.

The shopkeeper mimes getting each item off the shelf and taking the money (possibly even getting the group to help count the pennies) before the customer returns to their place. This process is repeated until everyone who wants to buy something from the shop does so. Jack doesn't necessarily have to buy beans if he doesn't want to, but lead someone to buy them eventually at the end of this section.

> **NOTE:** I have included the giant appearing as it is a good introduction to the character, but this mini-scene can be cut if necessary.

Routledge
Taylor & Francis Group

SHOPKEEPER: Uh oh. Here comes the giant.

GIANT: Fee! Fi! Fo! Fum!

Everyone hides, stays completely still or makes no noise while the giant is in the shop. The shopkeeper is very scared.

SHOPKEEPER: What would you like to buy?

GIANT: [item]

SHOPKEEPER: Would you like a big [item] or a small [item]?

GIANT: [response]

The shopkeeper mimes getting the giant's item. The giant then leaves and everyone can come back out of hiding.

SHOPKEEPER: Phew! That was close. Thank you everyone for coming to my shop. Please come again.

The shop is packed away while the participants return to their places, repeating the travelling song or playing the 'Follow-the-Leader' game.

Scene III: The Beanstalk

MUM: Welcome home. What did you buy at the shop Jack?

Mum can also ask everyone what he or she bought at the shop before getting to Jack.

JACK: I bought some magic beans.

ALL: Magic beans!

> **NOTE:** Guide the participants into saying 'Magic beans' by repeating and demonstrating this section of the script as many times as necessary.

MUM: Magic beans! We can't eat *them*.

Should the participants reply that the beans are edible, try one and screw up your face to show how awful it is before continuing.

MUM: I'm going to throw them out the window.

Count each bean as it is thrown out of the window.

MUM: Now go to bed!

The group returns to their original places to yawn, stretch and close their eyes.

NARRATOR: Overnight a beanstalk grew.

The group sings the 'When I Grow Up Song' (see the Explanation of Activities chapter).

NARRATOR: When Jack woke up he looked out of the window.

JACK: Wow! A beanstalk. Let's see what's at the top.

MUM: Be careful Jack.

They all climb the beanstalk (see 'Rope Walk' in the Explanation of Activities chapter).

Scene IV: The Giant's Kingdom

NARRATOR: Once they arrive at the top of the beanstalk the Giant's servant greets them.

> **NOTE:** As the shopkeeper character had an apron, give the servant a hat, since having another apron could confuse the group.

SERVANT: Hi! I'm the Giant's servant. Did you just climb up the beanstalk?

ALL: Yes.

> **NOTE:** This question can also be addressed to each individual, for example '[name] did you just climb up the beanstalk?' If the response is 'No', continue by asking participants where they came from and accept their answers.

SERVANT: Have you heard about the Giant? He's big. He's huge. He's MONSTROUS! If he comes, you need to run away and hide over here. Shall we practise?

> **NOTE:** 'Shall we practise?' is an important question as it allows you to demonstrate to the group what you need them to do, it gives participants the confidence to tackle the next stage of the drama, and allows some of them the opportunity to opt out if the drama is becoming too scary. They can observe from their chairs or the mats. Be specific and demonstrate exactly where you want the group to run to, otherwise they will disperse all over the room. If leading the drama in performance, change the wording to help guide the cast, for example, 'What do we do if the Giant comes Mr/Mrs Servant? Where shall we run to?', etc. Practise as many times as necessary.

SERVANT: So when the Giant comes, he says this ... Fee! Fi! Fo! Fum! ...

Practise this with the Giant.

SERVANT: ... and we run over here.

When everyone has practised running away, the Servant says the following rhyme, signalling to the giant for his entrance.

> *Giants, giants, everywhere*
> *If you see one please take care.*
> *Some are tall and some are fat*
> *Some are quiet as a cat.*
> *They pick their nose and suck their thumbs.*
> *Uh oh. Look out! Here one comes ...*

The Giant enters.

GIANT: *Fee! Fi! Fo! Fum!*
I smell the blood of an Englishman.
Be he alive or be he dead
I'll grind his bones to make my bread!

As the Giant appears, everyone runs and hides just as they had practised. The Giant then leaves.

SERVANT: Phew! That was close.

The above rhyme, running and hiding process can be repeated as often as you want before the Giant says his next line.

GIANT: Goose! Where are you Goose?

GOOSEY: Here I am.

Routledge
Taylor & Francis Group

> **NOTE:** Should the Giant forget this interaction, the script can skip straight to Goosey's 'Hello I'm Goosey' entrance. The role of Goosey can be cast from the group, stopping the action and guiding as mentioned. The character can then wear a feather boa, carry a feather duster or use a bird puppet.

GIANT: Where are my golden eggs?

GOOSEY: I'll go and get them.

GIANT: Don't try and steal them.

GOOSEY: I won't.

The Giant leaves and Goosey turns to the group.

GOOSEY: Hello. I'm Goosey. I work for the Giant. I lay his golden eggs. Have you ever seen a golden egg? Would you like one?

Goosey gets out a golden egg.

GOOSEY: Be careful with it. If you drop it the Giant will come back and take it.

Practise and reiterate these instructions. Should the Giant come back, there can be some further dialogue.

GIANT: Were you trying to steal the eggs Goose?

GOOSEY: No.

GIANT: I hope not.

The Giant takes back one of the eggs before leaving.

GOOSEY: That Giant is scary.

Scene V: Escaping Home

SERVANT: I know a way out of here. There's a secret passage behind the chimney, but we have to run under the fire.

> **NOTE:** Continue to guide the dialogue with cues such as 'Does anyone know a way out of here?' The workshop script is flexible and, even in performance, if lines are forgotten or the group gets off track, prompt with feeder lines, for example 'What is this story about? Does it have a beanstalk in it? Would you like to tell me about it? Can I tell them [the audience] about it?', etc.

Everyone does a 'Parachute Run' to escape the Giant's kingdom, including Goosey and the servant. Once everyone has escaped through the chimney, the plot continues.

NARRATOR: Here comes the Giant!

Incorporate a drum beat to match each chopping action as it helps to build tension.

ALL: Chop, chop, chop!

Repeat the 'Chop, chop, chop!', starting quietly and gaining in volume and height with each 'chop', until eventually the whole group is standing up.

NARRATOR: The Giant fell to the ground.

The participants all fall down.

NARRATOR: ... and everyone lived happily ever after.

End with a curtain call, where some lively music is playing and each participant comes forward to bow or curtsey.

JACK AND THE BEANSTALK

A SENSORY WORKSHOP

An example of tactile storytelling for those with profound and multiple learning difficulties (PMLD).

Character List

Narrator

Jack

Daisy the Cow

Market Man

Mum

Giant

Hen

Props List

- Jack's hat or costume
- Suede or leather material and/or a cowbell
- Some milk to drink
- Bag of magic beans (jelly beans or small beanbags)
- A jack-in-the-box or cone pop-up puppet (optional)
- A blanket to tuck the group into bed (optional)
- Shawl for mum
- A beanstalk (made from long strips of material fastened to a piece of dowelling with large cardboard leaves and shiny beans made from tinfoil)

> **NOTE:** If there is no time to make a beanstalk, a long roll of bubble-wrap can work just as well.

- Alarm clock noise
- Music for the growing beanstalk and escaping the Giant. (Suggestion: Grieg's *In the Hall of the Mountain King*)
- Feathers or bird puppet for hen
- Xylophone
- A drum (to make the sound for the Giant)
- Golden eggs (hard-boiled and sprayed with gold paint)
- A collection of big and small props, for example, shoes, baby clothes, large shirts, etc.
- Containers of cornflakes

Routledge
Taylor & Francis Group

WORKSHOP SCRIPT

Scene 1: Introducing Jack

Sing the 'Jack-in-the-Box' Rhyme (see the Explanation of Activities chapter), with everyone stretching their arms up high or using a real jack-in-the-box.

NARRATOR: Hello [name]. Do you know the story of 'Jack and the Beanstalk'?

Repeat the question to each participant as necessary.

NARRATOR: Well, Jack and his mum were very hungry.

Spend some time exploring 'empty' and 'full', for example, empty bowls, sparse contents of cereal packets, drink bottles, biscuit wrappers, etc. Listen to the sounds of full and empty containers when shaken and feel their weight. You could even count out cornflakes individually, saying, 'We've only got three cornflakes to eat' before saying the following rhyme.

NARRATOR: [name] Are you hungry, hungry, hungry?
                 [name] Are you hungry? I am too!

Repeat as necessary before taking on the role of Jack.

JACK: Hello [name]. I'm Jack and this is my cow Daisy.

Rub leather or suede material across the participants' faces or hands. 'Moo' and use a cowbell to signal Daisy.

JACK: We're off to the market. I have to sell Daisy to buy some food.

More 'moos' from Daisy and repeat to each participant as necessary.

JACK: I don't want to sell Daisy. She's my friend. She gives me milk. Would you like some milk?

Spend time drinking some milk and possibly trying other dairy products.

JACK: Oh well, come on Daisy. We'd better go to market.

Scene II: The Marketplace

Different sense of scene needed, either with background noise or a change of lighting in the room, while saying the following rhyme.

> *Jack is off to market, market, market.*
> *Jack is off to market, let's go too!*

After exploring the market for a while (an activity that could include smelling different types of food or trying on different types of clothes), Jack continues the story.

JACK: [name] Do you think someone here might like to buy my cow? I've been at this market a long time now and no one wants to buy her.

MARKET MAN: I'll buy her!

> **NOTE:** If there is just one person leading the drama, change role by saying, 'Someone over there is pointing to me. He looks like he works for the market. Shall I go and see what he wants? Can you [name] look after Daisy for me while I go and bring the Market Man over?' Dress the participant in charge of Daisy in Jack's costume and (if available) use an electronic communication device to help interaction between the newly cast Jack and the Market Man. Use any option available to encourage personal involvement by the participants and to prevent a common mistake of simply performing the story *at* the group.

MARKET MAN: Well hello Jack/[name]. I'd like to buy your cow. She's a beautiful cow and I'd like to give you something special for her ...

Repeat the dialogue and reiterate the cow's texture and sound.

MARKET MAN: ... some magic beans.

JACK: Magic beans?

Give the magic beans to Jack and take away Daisy (the leather material or cowbell).

> **NOTE:** To include the group further in this transaction, drop role and add dialogue such as '[name] Did you hear that? He wants to give Jack some magic beans for Daisy the Cow. Should he take them?' Alternatively, comment after the transaction has occurred, such as 'Did you sell Daisy? What did you get for her? Is this it? They're beans! It says on the side, "Magic beans". [name], you sold Daisy the Cow for some magic beans?', etc.

Routledge
Taylor & Francis Group

JACK: I don't know what Mum's going to say. We'd better head back home now.

The market background noise fades and the lights return for the change of scene.

Scene III: The Beanstalk

Mum enters.

MUM: So, there you all are! How was the market? Did you sell the cow? What's this? Beans? Magic beans?

Mum picks up the bag of magic beans and can even count them out.

MUM: [name], did you sell my cow for some magic beans? We can't eat magic beans! I'm going to throw them out of the window.

Each bean is thrown out of the window on the count of three, with music and crashing symbols to help signal the throw.

MUM: Now everyone. It's been a long day, so go to sleep.

The lights are turned off as the participants are helped to yawn, stretch and tucked into bed with a blanket. They can even play 'Snore Sshh!' (see the Explanation of Activities chapter). While the group is sleeping, the beanstalk is placed on the ground. The alarm clock sound (or a cock-a-doodle-doo) then wakes up the group as the lights come back on and Jack re-enters.

JACK: What a good night's sleep. I'm sorry mum didn't like the beans. What's this?

Jack points to the beanstalk material on the floor.

JACK: [name], do you know what this is? Shall we find out?

Jack slowly lifts the beanstalk high in the air.

JACK: Wow! A giant beanstalk. Look [name], a giant beanstalk. Shall we climb it?

     Shall we climb the beanstalk, beanstalk, beanstalk?
     Shall we climb the beanstalk to the sky?

The music for climbing the beanstalk starts as the beanstalk material is wrapped and wafted around each participant.

JACK: We made it!

Scene IV: The Giant's Kingdom

Another change of scene needed, achieved either with background noise, a change of lighting in room, or smells.

JACK: Look at this amazing place. Everything is really big.

Explore large and small props, for example different size balls, shoes, cups, etc. Spend time sorting big clothes from small to develop the Giant's character. Suddenly we hear a slow, deep drum sound.

JACK: What's that sound? Quick everyone, let's hide.

> **NOTE:** Either dress a participant up as the Giant, giving him the drum sound responsibility or, while hiding as Jack, change into the character of the Giant. However, if the character of the Giant or the drumbeat are too upsetting for some participants, cut out the Giant completely and go straight to the goose, golden eggs and home.

GIANT: *Fee! Fi! Fo! Fum!*
I smell the blood of an Englishman.
Be he alive or be he dead
I'll grind his bones to make my bread!

The Giant exits and Jack re-enters.

JACK: Who was that? He was huge. [name], did you see him? He must live here. I hope he doesn't come back.

The Giant can come back as often as necessary before Jack finds the golden eggs.

JACK: Phew! That was close. Hey, look at this. I've found a golden egg. [name], look what I've found, a golden egg. I wonder where it came from? Shall I go and have a look? [name], can you look after my golden egg for me?

Jack exits as Hen enters, greeting everyone by name and brushing feathers across their faces and/or arms.

HEN: Brrraaagghh! Hello. I see you've found a golden egg. I lay them you know. The Giant's always taking them, but I know a way to put the giant to sleep.

Repeat to each participant as necessary.

HEN: Just play this instrument.

Hen demonstrates playing the xylophone.

HEN: So, if the Giant comes back, just play this instrument and he'll fall asleep. Uh oh, here he comes.

The drumbeat returns to signal the Giant's entrance.

GIANT: Where are my eggs?

The xylophone music is played and the Giant falls asleep. He can wake up and be put to sleep many times before Jack re-enters.

Scene V: Escaping Home

JACK: Quick everyone, the Giant is fast asleep. Let's climb back down the beanstalk. Don't forget the golden eggs.

Let's climb down the beanstalk, beanstalk, beanstalk
Let's climb down the beanstalk and go home!

The beanstalk music starts again as the beanstalk is wafted back over the participants. Suddenly, the drumbeat starts.

JACK: Oh no. The Giant's woken up. Quick everyone, let's chop down the beanstalk.

As Jack says 'Chop, chop, chop!' over the music, the beanstalk gets smaller and smaller, eventually returning to a crumple of material on the floor. As this happens the drumbeat and the music become louder until on the final 'CHOP' everything is silent. Jack whispers to the participants.

JACK: I think we've done it.

Jack repeats it, getting louder.

JACK: I think we've done it. [name], we've escaped the Giant. And look at all this gold. We're rich. We can have loads of food now!

End the play with a feast.

Additional games and activities for either workshop

- Extend the marketplace scene by including animals and a farmer's market (see 'Animal Snap Cards' in the Explanation of Activities chapter). What else might you find at a market?

- Expand on the group going to sleep by singing a lullaby or ask the participants what they are dreaming about.

- Create the Giant's house with large cardboard plates or a giant door-frame, or discover what small things look like through a magnifying glass.

- Play 'Walking Around The Room As' (see the Explanation of Activities chapter).

- The Giant can order his servant around, which allows the group to play the 'Clean-Up Mime' (as in the 'Baboushka' workshop breakdown).

- Actually grow some beansprouts or other plants.

- Add an extra epilogue scene where Daisy the Cow returns to Jack at the end of the play.

Routledge
Taylor & Francis Group

EXPLANATION OF ACTIVITIES

Included in this chapter are descriptions of the various activities mentioned throughout the book, as well as a collection of games that can 'top and tail' any drama session, or be used as stand-alone time-fillers.

Animal snap cards

A collection of cards with different pairs of animals on them. These cards can be used in a variety of ways.

Find a friend

Give out the cards and ask members of the group to think about how their particular animal might move, what sound it might make, etc. Ask the participants (one at a time) to act out or show their particular animal to the rest of the group members, who must study their own cards to see if they are a match. If so, they can start to act with the other animal before sitting together as friends.

Pet shop or zoo trip

Use the cards for each participant to choose which animal they would like to buy, or visit, or feed. In pairs, one participant could be the animal, while the other could be the carer or zoo keeper. (Alternatively, have the group play different animals with you in role as the zoo keeper or pet store owner). Discover what types of food that particular animal might like to eat, or, if in a zoo, how big a pen it needs.

Freeze as

Play some appropriate music (I like to try and match the music to the theme of the workshop) for the group to dance to, and when the music stops someone chooses a card and the whole group must act like that particular animal until the music starts again.

Routledge Taylor & Francis Group   P   This page may be photocopied for instructional use only. Drama Scripts for People with Special Needs © Sheree Vickers 2005

Follow-the-leader

The group forms a line. The first person is the leader, choosing an animal card and starting to move as that particular animal. The rest of the group must follow, doing the same movements. When they have finished, ask the group what animal they thought was being represented before changing the leader of the group and choosing another animal card.

> **NOTE:** Although animal snap cards can be bought in various shops, they are easily made with cardboard and clip-art. Picture-pairs of people in various jobs or wearing cultural costumes can also be used with these games, or replace with characters from the various scripts, for example the Giant, Goosey, or the Postman.

Balloon tricks

Balloons are a wonderful prop and the different types of balloons available allow for various activities.

Punching bag

A big, thick party balloon is ideal for using as a punching bag.

> **NOTE:** In one particular group looking at bullying, I played a bear who was always looking for a fight and we used the balloon punching bag to illustrate this.

Keeping in the air

The object of this activity is to keep a blown-up a balloon in the air by tapping it. Count how many times the balloon is tapped to keep it afloat and try to beat this number.

Set up a competition with partners tapping to each other or use different coloured balloons for different teams. This is a wonderful game to promote teamwork.

Passing under legs or over heads

Play this game as one group, or in teams. Get the participants to line up behind each other. Blow a whistle and time how long it takes to pass the balloon down the line, either through their legs or over their heads (or alternating up and down).

Letting go fizzle

Blow the balloon up, don't tie it, hold it high, let it go and watch it fizzle around the room. Extend by having members of the group run after the balloon as it fizzles.

> **NOTE:** I first used this fizzle activity in a workshop where we had to learn to fly. This then led into a discussion on different modes of flying (from birds, to magic carpets, to aeroplanes). We then played 'Keeping In The Air', which eventually led the group to decide that if we filled ourselves up with air, we could float!

Squeaky sounds

Blow the balloon up and slowly squeak the air out of it. This creates a wonderfully funny sound that can be used for springing leaks in boats or creating character voices – I have actually had a discussion with a squeaky balloon who gave us clues to help us learn to fly (see above)!

Water bombs

Fill up some balloons with water, hold them high and watch them drop. (An activity best done outside.) They make a marvellous sound when they burst and create a wonderfully textured experience. Experiment with various sizes of balloons and amounts of water.

> **NOTE:** Before using any balloon tricks I always double-check whether any members of the group are particularly nervous of loud noises as there is always a chance of the balloon popping, and also if there are any participants with sensitive skin or latex allergies.

Clean-up mime

Make a list of clean-up activities, such as sweeping the floor, polishing the windows, vacuuming the carpets, and so forth. Randomly call out each activity and the group must then mime that action. Extend this game by locating each different clean-up activity in a different corner of the room. (See the 'Compass Game' for further explanation.)

Routledge
Taylor & Francis Group

This mime activity can be extended by having members of the group choose the action they enjoy doing the most before getting them to perform it individually to each other.

If using this game to begin each drama session, the group might want to show an activity they were doing earlier in the day, such as eating dinner, watching television or riding their bikes.

Compass game

A picture of a compass with the points (north, south, east and west) marked on it. These points correspond to points in the room that you demonstrate, for example 'When I call 'North' everyone runs to [here]', etc. (If necessary, mark each particular point with a mat or other visual aid.) You then call out the points in a random order and the group must gather in that particular location.

This game can be expanded by adding an activity that must be done in each particular area, for example North – jumping up and down, South – lie down and close your eyes, etc.

Alternatively, replace north, south, east and west with other points of reference, for example draw a map of the neighbourhood with Post Office, School, Laundry, Supermarket and various activities that correspond with those places.

Copy mime circle

Gather the group members into a circle, play some gentle music and move your arms, face and body (depending on the mobility of the group) while everyone copies your actions.

Pass the leadership of the movement on to somebody else so that the group then follows that person's actions. If necessary, run a commentary of the movements for those with visual impairments, for example '[name] is now moving his arms above his head and gently waving his fingers'. Eventually bring the mime back to yourself to finish the game.

Delivering the mail

Everyone is sitting on chairs. Three different items need to be delivered – a letter, a package and a telegram. If you call out 'letter', then the participants must all swap seats by walking. If you call out 'package', they must swap seats by crawling. If you call out 'telegram', they must swap seats by running.

If chairs are not possible, or you are concerned about safety when the group is running about, have them all sitting on a mat and, in small groups, deliver the letter, package or telegram to a postbox at one end of the room.

Adapt or extend this game by adding airmail, delivering by train, boat, or even travelling by donkey.

To complicate the game further, divide the names of three countries or cities between the group, so that whenever that particular country or city is called, only those participants may swap seats.

Don't move until I say ...

A favourite game of mine and groups that I work with. Originally I used the word 'monster', but any word can be used.

Play some music for the group to dance to. When the music stops the participants must 'freeze' and they are not allowed to move again until you say the appropriate word (in this case 'monster'). Have fun tricking them with all manner of 'M' words before saying the one needed. (Lead into or demonstrate this game a few times first, 'So if I say the word [music], can you move? If I say the word [mountain], can you move? But what if I say the word *monster* – can you move?').

To expand on this game, add a chase element in which, once the word is said, the participants must run back to their chairs or mats without being caught.

> **NOTE:** I guarantee that 'M' words will fail to come to mind when in the swing of this particular game, so keep a dictionary handy!

Routledge
Taylor & Francis Group

Flour sneeze

Sneezes are always fun and by adding some flour to your hand and blowing the sneeze into it, a lovely texture and visual image is created. This also helps to define location, for example a bakery in 'My Neighbourhood' or even as cement, if on a building site in 'Training Day'.

Grandmother's footsteps

The traditional game is played by having someone as Grandma turn their back or close their eyes as the rest of the group (or an individual) tries to sneak up on them. When Grandma turns around or opens her eyes, the sneaking group must freeze. Anyone caught moving is sent back to the start line. If the participants eventually manage to reach Grandma, she is tagged and must then chase the group back to the start line. If anyone is caught, they become Grandma.

This game can easily be adapted for different characters, for example a police officer sneaking up on a burglar (as in 'My Neighbourhood'), a knight sneaking up on a dragon (as in 'Dragon Sleep') or a postman sneaking up on a scary dog (see 'Training Day').

I went to the shop

This is a traditional memory game. Say the rhyme, 'I went to the shop and I bought a [apple]', naming something you might buy. When the next person says the rhyme they must also repeat your item. Slowly the shopping list gets longer and longer. The first person might buy an apple, the next person buys an apple and a teddy bear, the next person buys an apple, a teddy bear and a pot plant, and so forth.

This is also a good game to adapt for learning people's names.

Jack-in-the-box rhyme

Traditional – to the tune of 'Here We Go Round the Mulberry Bush'. Start this rhyme crouching down, ready to jump up and wave your arms in the air before pushing yourself back down again. (If you can find a big enough box, have fun decorating it and jumping out of that!)

Jack-in-the-Box jumps up like this.
He makes me laugh as he waggles his head.
I gently press him down again,
Saying 'Jack-in-the-Box you must go to bed!'

Karate chop duck

In character as Master Karate Expert, and using a pretend sword or stick, give the group the following instructions (with appropriate Kung Fu-type noises):

When I swing my sword low [action of bobbing down and swinging imaginary sword or stick] *you all jump up high.*

When I swing my sword high [action of stretching up high and swinging imaginary sword or stick] *you all duck down low.*

Practise, demonstrate, extend or simplify the actions or characters.

NOTE: If the participants are in wheelchairs, replace standing up with putting your arms in the air and ducking down with putting your hands on your head. They can also be assisted with this if necessary.

Musical statues sshoosh

The group dances to loud music. When the music gets switched off, the participants freeze as a grumpy old character (such as Mama if using for 'My Neighbourhood') enters and tells them to turn the music down because it's too loud. When she exits the music and dancing recommence. End the activity when the music ends.

NOTE: Older participants love interacting with the grumpy old character (who is more comical than scary) and an improvised dialogue occasionally happens.

This game can also be played as musical chairs or bobs. When the music stops, the participants must return to their chairs or mats, or sit down on the floor.

Routledge
Taylor & Francis Group

As a further adaptation, replace the music with participants making a lot of noise, for example sitting in a classroom waiting for the teacher to arrive. When the teacher character appears, the group must return instantly to their places, acting innocent and staying quiet until she leaves again.

Opening meet and greet song or goodbye song

To the tune of *Frère Jacques*. A lovely way to use this song is with a shared hat and instrument. Whoever is being sung to by the group can wear the hat and use the instrument, but must then pass it on to the next person. It is important that the hat and instrument are given to the next person by the previous participant, to reiterate that drama is a shared endeavour.

> *Hello* [name] ... Hello [name]
> *How are you?* ... How are you?
> *It's very nice to meet you!* ... It's very nice to meet you!
> *Let's have fun!* ... Let's have fun!
>
> *Goodbye* [name] ... Goodbye [name]
> *See you soon* ... See you soon.
> *It's been good to meet you* ... It's been good to meet you.
> *Bye for now.* ... Bye for now.

NOTE: Personally I'm not very confident with song, so when inventing this song to use in my drama lessons, I stuck to a tune I knew well. (I use *Frère Jacques* a lot.)

Parachute runs

Two people hold each end of a long piece of material and either waft it over each participant, or, as the material soars up, on the count of three each member of the group (individually or in pairs) must run under it.

NOTE: I love the 'Parachute Runs': from using blue material for the waves of the sea, or bright red material for escaping a fiery dragon, to using netting to escape fishermen, or creating a magical glittery entrance for a Cinderella ball.

Rope walk

Lay a rope on the ground for the participants to walk along as accurately as possible. It may be in a straight line or all higgledy-piggledy along the floor. Demonstrate how to do it first (it is not as easy as you might think)!

This activity can be used to climb the beanstalk (see the 'Jack and the Beanstalk' workshop breakdown) or for a tightrope walker in the circus, or to create a treacherous jungle walk!

Run away boo!

An adaptation of 'Grandmother's Footsteps' (see earlier description), except that the character of the Ghost is hidden behind a curtain or around a corner. Individually, or in pairs, participants sneak up, knock on the door or say 'Hello, anyone home?' and wait for the Ghost to say 'Boo!', before running away scared back to their places.

Change the character of the Ghost and what it says to suit the script, for example the Giant in 'Jack and the Beanstalk', Banquo in 'Macbeth', or the Dragon in 'Dragon Sleep'.

Sailor went to sea song

A sailor went to sea sea sea
To see what he could see see see
And all that he could see see see
Was the bottom of the deep blue sea sea sea

Snore sshh!

The group is very quiet, trying to get to sleep. Someone is tapped on the head and he or she has to snore very loudly. The rest of the group then have to go 'Sshh!' before all is silent again.

Adapt this game by having the participants make all sorts of different sounds, such as animal noises, coughs, sneezes, etc.

Routledge Taylor & Francis Group

Sound orchestra

Using instruments and a conductor, explore loud and quiet sounds with the visual cue of the conductor standing up with arms high in the air (for loud) and crouching down very small (for quiet). Practise with individuals before slowly adding more and more people to create a group orchestra.

Replace the instruments with sounds you can make with your body, such as clapping hands and raspberry-blowing lips, or create a menagerie of sounds for different scenes, such as animals, the ocean, or people in the neighbourhood.

Ten brown teddies

To the tune of *Ten Green Bottles.*

> *Ten brown teddies, sitting on the wall,*
> *Ten brown teddies, sitting on the wall,*
> *And if one brown teddy went to the shopping mall …*

Spend some time discovering, via questions, mime and props, what the participants might buy at the shopping mall before continuing with the song.

> *… There'll be nine brown teddies, sitting on the wall.*

When I grow up song

To the tune of *Frère Jacques.* Sing the song and ask each participant what they would like to be when they grow up. Extend this further by getting them to mime what they want to be, while the rest of the group tries to guess what it is.

> *When I grow up …* When I grow up
> *I will be …* I will be
> *Anything I want to …* Anything I want to
> *Wait and see …* Wait and see

Walking around the room as ...

With the group, walk around the room as various characters are called out at random. Using 'Jack and the Beanstalk' as an example, walk around the room as a Giant, as Daisy the Cow, as Mum, as the Servant, as Goosey, as Jack etc.

Don't forget to remind the participants that faces are very important. This game can be extended, for example 'Show me Jack walking around very scared. What is something he might say if he is very scared?', etc.

> **NOTE:** If mobility is a problem, just use the faces part of this exercise with a mirror to help participants show an angry face or a happy face, etc. Often, with PMLD groups, I have also associated a sound with each emotional face.

Wash rinse spin stop

Call out each of the following actions in a random order:

- On 'Wash', the participants mime the action of washing their faces, legs and arms.
- On 'Rinse', tinkle fingers down like rain.
- On 'Spin', turn in a circle.
- On 'Stop', they freeze or sit down.

Combine this activity with musical chairs and add an 'overload' command. When 'Overload' is called, everyone must rush out of the washing machine, back to his or her original place. The last one back to his seat is out.

To create a more sensory activity, blow some bubbles over the group, add some confetti soap powder and use a water mist spray.

Who's got the jewels?

The participants sit either in a circle or in a line. A volunteer (the detective or police officer) leaves the room as a bag of costume jewels are secretly given to another member of the group (the burglar). When the detective re-enters, the burglar must carefully and secretly start passing the bag of jewels along the line of participants without being caught. Encourage the participants to be sneaky and pass the jewels behind their backs. It is up to the detective to catch the thief.

> **NOTE:** The burglar is caught only by the jewels being seen. The detective may not 'frisk' the burglar or make contact with him in any way.

If working with a group with more profound learning difficulties, dress the burglar up and when the detective re-enters he must look closely to discover who is wearing the costume jewels.

Adapt this game for 'Dragon Sleep' and stealing the jewels away from the Dragon, or for pirates finding treasure, or even stealing a biscuit from a biscuit tin.

*For Product Safety Concerns and Information please contact
our EU representative GPSR@taylorandfrancis.com Taylor & Francis
Verlag GmbH, Kaufingerstraße 24, 80331 München, Germany*

T - #0005 - 160425 - C0 - 297/210/8 - SB - 9780863885297 - Gloss Lamination